INTERMITTENT FASTING FOR HORMONAL BALANCE IN WOMEN OVER 50

Science-backed Strategies for PMS Relief, Perimenopause Harmony, & Weight Management + Meal Plans & Recipes for Hormone-Balancing Success

Robert Maverick

Copyright © 2023

by

Robert Maverick

Disclaimer: The information in this book is for general informational purposes only and should not be considered as professional advice. The author and publisher disclaim any liability arising directly or indirectly from the use of this information.

Table of Contents

Introduction

In the vibrant tapestry of a woman's life, navigating the intricate dance of hormones becomes an essential rhythm, especially as we gracefully embrace the golden era of our fifties. Welcome to "Intermittent Fasting for Hormonal Balance in Women Over 50" is a complete guide for adult women looking for balance in the throes of perimenopause, PMS, and the always changing world of weight control.

Embarking on this journey is an empowering choice, a commitment to understanding and embracing the incredible nuances of your body. As we delve into the heart of this guide, envision a roadmap curated with scientific precision and adorned with the compassionate wisdom that acknowledges the unique needs of women over 50.

This isn't just a book; it's a lifeline for those seeking relief from the capricious dance of hormones. You'll discover the transformative power of intermittent fasting, a science-backed strategy that unfolds as a key to unlocking hormonal equilibrium. With each turn of the page, you'll find not only the why but also the how, as we unravel the intricate web of hormonal intricacies with accessible explanations and relatable insights.

Picture this as your personal sanctuary, a space where knowledge transforms into action. Science and strategy intertwine seamlessly, offering practical tools for PMS relief, perimenopause harmony, and weight management tailored specifically for the needs of women navigating the golden chapter of life.

But it doesn't stop there — within these pages, you'll uncover more than just information. Expect to be embraced by delicious meal plans and easy recipes designed not only to nourish your body but to elevate your spirit. This isn't about restriction; it's about celebration — celebrating the wisdom your body holds and providing it with the sustenance it deserves.

As you immerse yourself in these empowering insights, know that you're not alone on this journey. Consider this book a supportive companion, offering understanding and encouragement as you make choices that resonate with the rhythm of your life. Your empowerment is our goal, and your success is the heartbeat of this narrative.

So, let's embark on this transformative adventure together. May each chapter be a stepping stone towards hormonal balance, a path illuminated by science, compassion, and the vibrant tapestry of your own strength. Welcome to a journey that transcends the pages — welcome to the thriving community of women championing hormonal harmony in their fifties and beyond.

The Importance of Hormonal Balance in Women Over 50

In the pages of **Intermittent Fasting for Hormonal Balance in Women Over 50**, a transformative journey unfolds, shedding light on the paramount significance of hormonal balance for women navigating the golden years of life. This empowering guide, woven with compassion and support, stands as a beacon for those seeking not just relief but a holistic approach to well-being.

As women embrace the milestone of 50 and beyond, the intricate dance of hormones within the body takes center stage. This book intricately explores the intricate web of hormonal fluctuations, offering science-backed strategies that extend a helping hand through the challenges of PMS, the nuances of perimenopause, and the quest for weight management.

Delving into the science behind intermittent fasting, the narrative unveils a tapestry of strategies meticulously designed to harmonize hormonal rhythms. With a focus on PMS relief, the book becomes a companion in the journey toward finding equilibrium during the transitional phase of perimenopause. It delicately acknowledges the unique experiences of women, providing not just information but a compassionate understanding of the changes unfolding within.

Weight management, another crucial facet, takes center stage, revealing the symbiotic relationship between hormonal balance and maintaining a healthy weight. Engagingly, the book navigates the intricacies of metabolism and body composition, fostering a sense of empowerment for women who aspire to take charge of their well-being.

Beyond the realm of information, "Intermittent Fasting for Hormonal Balance in Women Over 50" extends its embrace with delectable meal plans and easy recipes. These culinary companions are crafted not just for nourishment but as tools for hormone-balancing success. The pages resonate with accessibility, ensuring that every woman, regardless of her culinary prowess, finds joy in preparing meals that cater to her hormonal harmony.

In this comprehensive guide, the narrative transcends the conventional boundaries of health literature. It becomes a testament to the strength, resilience, and beauty that accompanies the journey of women over 50. Rooted in science, enriched with compassion, and adorned with practicality, this book stands as a beacon, illuminating the path toward hormonal balance, vitality, and a thriving journey through the remarkable years that lie ahead.

As the pages unfold, the narrative weaves a tapestry of empowerment, urging women over 50 to embrace their bodies as allies, navigating the ebb and flow of hormonal shifts with grace and understanding. The storytelling takes a turn toward the practical, offering a roadmap for implementing intermittent fasting as a sustainable lifestyle choice.

With an understanding that every woman's journey is unique, the book provides not just a one-size-fits-all approach but a personalized guide. The reader is gently encouraged to listen to her body's whispers, honoring its signals and responding with kindness. It becomes a journey of self-discovery, where the power to balance hormones is not imposed but discovered within.

The discussion on perimenopause is handled with a delicate touch, acknowledging the challenges that may arise. From mood swings to sleep disturbances, the narrative becomes a companion, assuring women that they are not alone in this transformative phase. The science-backed strategies presented serve as tools of resilience, aiding in the creation of a harmonious balance that extends beyond the physiological realm.

The emphasis on PMS relief goes beyond offering mere solutions; it becomes a celebration of the resilience inherent in every woman. The book not only provides insights into managing symptoms but instills a sense of pride in the ability to navigate through the monthly cycles with strength and poise.

The journey of weight management takes center stage, not as a quest for societal ideals but as a pursuit of individual well-being. The narrative dismantles stereotypes, fostering a culture of body positivity and self-love. It encourages women to view their bodies not as battlegrounds but as allies in the pursuit of a vibrant and fulfilling life.

The meal plans and recipes woven into the narrative are not just about sustenance; they become rituals of self-care. With simplicity at their core, these culinary offerings are designed to make the journey enjoyable and accessible. The book unfolds a world where nourishment is not a chore but a celebration, inviting women to savor the joy of balancing hormones through delightful and satisfying meals.

In the final chapters, the narrative circles back to the heart of the matter—the celebration of women over 50 embracing a life rich in vitality, wisdom, and self-love. It leaves readers not just with knowledge but with a sense of camaraderie, reminding them that the journey through hormonal balance is not a solitary one but a collective dance of strength, resilience, and empowerment.

Brief Overview of Intermittent Fasting as a Tool for Hormonal Health

In the realm of women's health and wellness, **Intermittent Fasting for Hormonal Balance in Women Over 50** serves as a beacon of empowerment and knowledge. This comprehensive guide navigates the intricate terrain of hormonal health, particularly catering to the unique needs of women at a pivotal stage in their lives.

The book opens with a compelling narrative, weaving together the science and personal stories that underscore the transformative potential of intermittent fasting. It demystifies the concept, revealing it not just as a weight management tool but as a powerful strategy for hormonal equilibrium. The language is accessible, ensuring that readers of all backgrounds can grasp the essential principles without feeling overwhelmed.

Delving into the core theme, the book explores how intermittent fasting becomes a reliable ally in the battle against the often-dreaded PMS symptoms. With a compassionate tone, it acknowledges the challenges many women face during this phase of life and provides science-backed strategies for relief. The narrative unfolds like a supportive friend, guiding readers through practical steps to navigate this hormonal rollercoaster with grace and resilience.

As the journey continues into the realm of perimenopause, the book maintains its informative and engaging style. It discusses the natural shifts in hormonal patterns, emphasizing how intermittent fasting can be a harmonizing force during this transformative period. The narrative refrains from portraying perimenopause as a stumbling block but rather as an opportunity for self-discovery and growth.

Weight management takes center stage, not as an elusive goal but as a natural outcome of the hormonal balance achieved through intermittent fasting. The book offers practical tips, delicious meal plans, and easy recipes that make the journey enjoyable and sustainable. It dismantles the notion of restrictive diets and fosters a positive relationship with food, encouraging readers to savor nourishing meals that support hormonal well-being.

Throughout the narrative, the author's voice resonates with empathy, understanding the diverse experiences women undergo. The book becomes a companion, addressing the concerns and questions that may arise on this transformative journey. The language remains uplifting, reinforcing the idea that embracing intermittent fasting is not just a health strategy but a celebration of a woman's innate strength and resilience.

In essence, offering a thorough yet approachable road map for ladies seeking treatment from PMS, "Intermittent Fasting for Hormonal Balance in Women Over 50" is a shining example of empowerment. perimenopausal harmony, and weight management. It is a testament to the profound impact of intermittent fasting on hormonal health and a guide that uplifts, informs, and supports women on their path to hormonal-balancing success.

Chapter 1
Understanding Hormonal Changes After 50

In this Chapter, we embark on a journey to unravel the intricate tapestry of hormonal changes that grace the stage of a woman's life after the age of 50. This pivotal chapter lays the foundation for understanding the physiological shifts that unfold, paving the way for a comprehensive approach to harnessing the power of intermittent fasting for hormonal equilibrium.

As a woman traverses the milestone of 50, her body undergoes a symphony of hormonal fluctuations. Estrogen, progesterone, and testosterone—the orchestrators of vitality—enter a new rhythm, often characterized by a gradual decline. This hormonal dance, while a natural progression, can manifest in a spectrum of symptoms, from the notorious hot flashes to mood swings and the intricacies of perimenopause.

Scientific research serves as our guiding beacon, shedding light on the nuanced ways in which intermittent fasting can be a transformative ally in navigating these hormonal waters. By embracing intermittent fasting, women over 50 may find relief from PMS symptoms, experience harmonious transitions through perimenopause, and even discover a companion in their journey towards weight management.

Delving deeper into the science, we explore how intermittent fasting triggers cellular responses, influencing gene expression and hormonal balance. The fasting periods initiate autophagy, a cellular "clean-up" process that holds promise in mitigating age-related changes. This not only aligns with the natural ebb and flow of hormones but also presents an opportunity for the body to recalibrate itself, fostering a renewed sense of well-being.

Our narrative seamlessly weaves in the challenges faced by women over 50, acknowledging the unique intersectionality of hormonal changes and the importance of tailored strategies. Empowering and informative, this chapter sets the stage for actionable insights, presenting intermittent fasting not as a mere dietary approach but as a lifestyle choice with profound implications for hormonal health.

To support our readers on this transformative journey, we introduce practical tips, personalized meal plans, and tantalizing recipes designed with the specific needs of women over 50 in mind. These are not just culinary delights; they are strategic tools in the pursuit of hormone-balancing success.

In essence, Chapter 1 serves as a compass, guiding women over 50 through the labyrinth of hormonal changes with wisdom, scientific backing, and a touch of culinary allure. It is an ode to resilience, a roadmap for empowerment, and an invitation to embrace the transformative potential of intermittent fasting for a harmonious and vibrant second act of life.

As we navigate the landscape of hormonal changes after 50, our journey extends beyond the scientific realm to embrace the emotional and psychological facets of this transformative phase. Chapter 1 recognizes that the hormonal symphony is not merely a physiological phenomenon; it is an integral part of a woman's identity and well-being.

With empathy as our compass, we delve into the emotional nuances of hormonal fluctuations. From the contemplative moments of self-discovery to the challenges that may arise, this chapter weaves a narrative that resonates with the lived experiences of women over 50. It acknowledges the resilience required to embrace change and provides a supportive space for navigating the intricacies of this chapter in life.

Understanding hormonal changes isn't just about decoding biological processes; it's about fostering a sense of community. Women over 50 are not alone in this journey, and this chapter aims to create a collective narrative, emphasizing shared experiences and shared wisdom. Through stories of triumph and vulnerability, readers find solace, knowing that they are part of a resilient sisterhood navigating similar waters.

In our quest for hormonal balance, actionable steps take center stage. Chapter 1 transforms knowledge into empowerment by offering practical strategies that women can integrate seamlessly into their lives. From personalized intermittent fasting schedules to mindful practices that enhance hormonal resilience, every recommendation is tailored to the unique needs of our audience.

As we embrace the science-backed strategies for PMS relief, perimenopause harmony, and weight management, the chapter unfolds like a personalized guide, offering not just information but a roadmap for implementation. Each woman is invited to embark on her own transformative journey, equipped with the knowledge and tools needed for success.

To further enhance the engagement of our readers, Chapter 1 introduces a dynamic interplay between information and interaction. From thought-provoking reflection prompts to opportunities for sharing personal insights, the narrative extends beyond the pages, fostering a sense of connection and active participation.

The chapter concludes with a promise—a promise of transformation, resilience, and empowerment. It sets the stage for the subsequent chapters, where the science-backed strategies introduced here will be woven into the fabric of delicious meal plans and easy recipes. The culinary journey becomes a celebration of both nourishment and joy, offering a tangible and delectable path toward hormonal balance.

In essence, Chapter 1 transcends the boundaries of conventional literature. It is not merely a chapter; it is an immersive experience—an exploration of science, emotion, and empowerment. It beckons women over 50 to embrace the beauty of their hormonal evolution and embark on a transformative odyssey towards a harmonious and vibrant second act of life.

Overview of Menopause and Perimenopause

In the intricate journey of a woman's life, the phases of menopause and perimenopause represent transformative chapters often accompanied by a spectrum of physical, emotional, and hormonal shifts. As we navigate the realms of hormonal balance in the golden years, it becomes imperative to delve into a comprehensive overview of menopause and perimenopause, tailored specifically for the resilient women over 50.

Understanding Menopause: A Metamorphic Transition

Menopause, a natural biological process, marks the cessation of menstrual cycles, typically occurring in a woman's late 40s to early 50s. This pivotal milestone heralds the conclusion of reproductive capabilities and brings forth a cascade of hormonal alterations, prominently the decline in estrogen and progesterone levels. The nuanced dance of hormones during menopause triggers a myriad of symptoms, ranging from hot flashes and night sweats to mood swings and changes in libido.

Engaging with our target audience, women over 50, it's essential to convey that this phase is not merely a cessation of fertility but a transformative journey requiring tailored self-care. Acknowledging and embracing the changes, both physical and emotional, is paramount to fostering a positive menopausal experience.

Perimenopause: The Prelude to Menopause

Preceding menopause, women traverse the realm of perimenopause, a transitional phase that typically begins in the late 30s or early 40s. During perimenopause, hormonal fluctuations intensify, leading to irregular menstrual cycles and an array of symptoms mirroring those of menopause. This stage is characterized by the ebb and flow of estrogen and progesterone, paving the way for the eventual decline in ovarian function.

Navigating perimenopause requires a nuanced approach, and as we connect with our audience, it's crucial to empower them with actionable insights. Educating women over 50 on the diverse manifestations of perimenopause, from mood swings to sleep disturbances, fosters a sense of understanding and resilience in the face of these changes.

Empowerment Through Knowledge: Navigating the Terrain

Arming oneself with knowledge becomes a potent tool for women over 50 navigating menopause and perimenopause. Recognizing that these changes are not just physical but also impact emotional well-being fosters a proactive approach to holistic health.

Scientifically backed strategies, such as intermittent fasting, can play a pivotal role in managing symptoms and supporting hormonal balance. Intermittent fasting has been shown to influence insulin sensitivity, promote fat loss, and mitigate some of the challenges associated with hormonal fluctuations.

In the subsequent chapters of our journey through "Intermittent Fasting for Hormonal Balance in Women Over

50," we'll delve deeper into actionable steps and explore how incorporating this approach into your lifestyle can provide relief from PMS symptoms, harmonize perimenopause, and aid in weight management.

Stay tuned as we unravel the mysteries, celebrate the strengths, and empower women over 50 to embrace this transformative phase with resilience, grace, and a commitment to holistic well-being. After all, menopause is not just an end; it's a compelling beginning – a gateway to a new era of self-discovery and vitality.

Scientific Backing for Hormonal Harmony

Our narrative extends beyond mere descriptions, incorporating a scientific foundation to empower women with knowledge. Exploring the scientific underpinnings of hormonal fluctuations during menopause and perimenopause equips our audience with a deeper understanding of their bodies. By elucidating the role of hormones in this journey, we foster an appreciation for the interconnectedness of lifestyle choices, hormonal balance, and overall well-being.

Common Hormonal Imbalances in Women Over 50

In the intricate tapestry of a woman's life, the onset of the fifties marks a significant chapter—a juncture where hormonal nuances can usher in a myriad of changes. As we embark on the exploration of "Common Hormonal Imbalances in Women Over 50" within the context of intermittent fasting for hormonal balance, let's navigate through the subtleties and intricacies that define this pivotal phase of life.

Estrogen Dominance: The delicate dance between estrogen and progesterone takes center stage during menopause, often leading to estrogen dominance. This imbalance can contribute to weight gain, mood swings, and disrupted sleep patterns.

Progesterone Deficiency: As menopause unfolds, progesterone levels decline, potentially causing irregular menstrual cycles, heightened stress responses, and a propensity for anxiety.

Thyroid Dysfunction: The thyroid, a conductor of the body's metabolic symphony, may undergo imbalances, resulting in fatigue, weight fluctuations, and a sense of mental fog—common concerns for women in their fifties.

Cortisol Irregularities: Elevated stress levels can disrupt cortisol production, impacting sleep quality, immune function, and exacerbating the challenges posed by hormonal fluctuations.

Insulin Resistance: The body's response to insulin may diminish with age, potentially leading to weight gain, particularly around the abdominal region, and an increased risk of developing type 2 diabetes.

Melatonin Disruption: Sleep disturbances become more prevalent with age, affecting melatonin production. This hormonal shift not only impacts sleep quality but can also influence mood and cognitive function.

DHEA Decline: Dehydroepiandrosterone (DHEA), a precursor to estrogen and testosterone, decreases with age, influencing energy levels, muscle mass, and overall vitality.

Testosterone Fluctuations: While often associated with men, testosterone plays a crucial role in women's health. Its decline can contribute to diminished libido, fatigue, and a decline in muscle mass.

Growth Hormone Reduction: The decline in growth hormone production can impede muscle maintenance, recovery, and overall vitality, making it crucial to address this hormonal shift.

Serotonin Imbalance: Serotonin, a neurotransmitter linked to mood regulation, may fluctuate, contributing to mood swings, irritability, and an increased susceptibility to anxiety and depression.

Corticotropin-Releasing Hormone (CRH) Fluctuations: Stress-related hormonal shifts involving CRH can impact various bodily functions, from digestion to immune response, necessitating a holistic approach to hormonal balance.

Vitamin D Insufficiency: Beyond its role in bone health, vitamin D deficiency can influence hormonal balance, potentially contributing to mood disorders and compromised immune function.

Leptin Resistance: Leptin, a hormone regulating appetite, may face resistance, leading to challenges in weight management and an increased risk of obesity.

Prolactin Variations: Elevated levels of prolactin, typically associated with lactation, can occur outside pregnancy, contributing to disruptions in the menstrual cycle and fertility.

Aldosterone Imbalance: This hormone, crucial for regulating blood pressure and electrolyte balance, may fluctuate, impacting cardiovascular health and overall well-being.

Adiponectin Reduction: A decline in adiponectin levels can affect insulin sensitivity and fat metabolism, playing a role in the development of metabolic syndrome.

Follicle-Stimulating Hormone (FSH) Surge: Menopause triggers a surge in FSH, impacting reproductive functions and contributing to symptoms like hot flashes and mood swings.

Gonadotropin-Releasing Hormone (GnRH) Changes: Alterations in GnRH levels can influence reproductive health, contributing to irregular menstrual cycles and other menopausal symptoms.

Renin-Angiotensin System (RAS) Fluctuations: Changes in RAS activity can impact blood pressure regulation, highlighting the interconnectedness of hormonal systems in the body.

Oxytocin Variability: Beyond its role in childbirth and bonding, oxytocin fluctuations can influence social interactions, stress responses, and emotional well-being during this phase of life.

As we delve into the intricacies of hormonal imbalances in women over 50, it becomes apparent that a multifaceted approach, integrating intermittent fasting with tailored lifestyle adjustments, holds the key to navigating this transformative journey with grace and vitality. Stay tuned as we unravel the science-backed strategies for PMS relief, perimenopausal harmony, and weight management, accompanied by delectable meal plans and recipes designed to support hormone-balancing success in the chapters to follow.

Impact of Hormones on PMS, Mood, and Weight Management

In the intricate tapestry of a woman's life, the impact of hormones transcends mere biological functions; it shapes the symphony of her well-being. For women over 50, this journey is often characterized by the delicate dance of hormones, influencing not just physical health but also mood and weight management. As we delve into the realm of hormonal fluctuations, exploring the profound relationship between hormones, PMS, mood, and weight becomes crucial on the path to holistic well-being.

Picture this: you're navigating the intricate labyrinth of perimenopause, a phase where hormonal shifts take center stage. Estrogen, progesterone, and testosterone, the hormonal trio orchestrating your body's intricate ballet, undergo fluctuations that can manifest in various ways. One prominent player in this hormonal narrative is estrogen, whose decline can lead to an array of symptoms, including the notorious PMS.

Understanding the impact of hormones on PMS for women over 50 is akin to deciphering the whispers of a language your body speaks. The rollercoaster of emotions, bloating, and irritability that accompany PMS can be attributed to the intricate hormonal interplay. Educating ourselves on this topic empowers us to navigate these fluctuations with resilience.

Equally significant is the sway hormones hold over mood during this life stage. Serotonin, often referred to as the "feel-good" neurotransmitter, experiences ebbs and flows influenced by hormonal changes. The result? Mood swings that can feel like emotional tidal waves. Acknowledging the connection between hormones and mood becomes a key step in reclaiming emotional harmony.

Now, let's unravel the weighty matter of weight management. Hormonal fluctuations, particularly the decrease in estrogen levels, can impact metabolism and lead to changes in body composition. As women over 50 embark on a journey to manage their weight, understanding the hormonal nuances becomes a compass guiding them through the terrain of effective strategies.

Scientifically backed insights pave the way for actionable steps tailored to the unique needs of women over 50. Incorporating intermittent fasting into the equation emerges as a promising strategy. Research suggests that intermittent fasting can positively influence hormonal balance, offering a beacon of hope for those seeking relief from PMS symptoms, mood swings, and weight management challenges.

Empowering women over 50 with science-backed strategies for hormonal balance is not merely an intellectual pursuit but a compassionate embrace of their unique journey. The narrative unfolds as a beacon of light, weaving together education, support, and actionable steps, all grounded in the bedrock of scientific understanding.

In this chapter of **Intermittent Fasting for Hormonal Balance in Women Over 50**, the journey of exploration extends beyond the confines of hormonal intricacies. It is a celebration of resilience, a testament to the strength inherent in every woman navigating the realms of perimenopause and beyond. The goal? To not just weather the hormonal storms but to emerge empowered, informed, and in harmony with the symphony of life after 50.

In the journey of embracing intermittent fasting for hormonal balance, understanding the profound impact hormones wield on various aspects of women's health becomes pivotal, especially for those navigating the vibrant landscape of their 50s. This chapter delves into the intricate dance between hormones, focusing on the 15 key facets that shape the experience of PMS, mood, and weight management for women over 50.

Estrogen Fluctuations and Mood Swings: As estrogen levels fluctuate during perimenopause, the delicate balance of neurotransmitters in the brain is affected, giving rise to mood swings and emotional turbulence.

Progesterone's Influence on Sleep Quality: Declining progesterone levels contribute to sleep disturbances, impacting overall well-being. Addressing sleep hygiene becomes paramount in managing hormonal fluctuations.

Insulin Sensitivity and Weight Management: Hormonal shifts can lead to insulin resistance, affecting how the body processes glucose. Intermittent fasting emerges as a powerful tool to enhance insulin sensitivity, aiding in weight management.

Cortisol and Stress Response: Elevated cortisol levels, often associated with stress, can exacerbate PMS symptoms. Strategies such as mindfulness and intermittent fasting prove beneficial in modulating cortisol responses.

Thyroid Function and Metabolism: Hormonal changes can influence thyroid function, impacting metabolism. Tailoring intermittent fasting approaches to support thyroid health is crucial for weight management.

Serotonin and Mood Regulation: Serotonin, a neurotransmitter linked to mood regulation, can be influenced by hormonal shifts. Intermittent fasting, combined with serotonin-boosting foods, supports a positive emotional state.

Leptin and Appetite Control: Fluctuations in leptin levels can disrupt appetite regulation. Intermittent fasting aids in restoring leptin sensitivity, promoting a healthier relationship with food.

Ghrelin's Role in Hunger Signals: Understanding ghrelin, the hunger hormone, is essential in crafting effective intermittent fasting plans. Balancing ghrelin levels contributes to better appetite control.

Melatonin for Sleep Quality: Hormonal changes impact melatonin production, affecting sleep quality. Incorporating intermittent fasting alongside melatonin-rich foods promotes restorative sleep.

DHEA and Energy Levels: Dehydroepiandrosterone (DHEA) levels decline with age, impacting energy levels. Intermittent fasting supports DHEA production, contributing to sustained vitality.

Aldosterone and Water Retention: Hormonal fluctuations can contribute to water retention. Intermittent fasting, coupled with hydration strategies, helps regulate aldosterone levels for optimal fluid balance.

Testosterone's Role in Lean Muscle Mass: Declining testosterone levels may lead to muscle loss. Intermittent fasting, complemented by resistance training, aids in preserving lean muscle mass.

Prolactin and Breast Health: Balancing prolactin levels through intermittent fasting aligns with promoting breast health, contributing to overall well-being during this life stage.

Catecholamines and Exercise Performance: Hormones like adrenaline impact exercise performance. Tailoring intermittent fasting around workout schedules optimizes the release of catecholamines, enhancing fitness outcomes.

Hormonal Harmony Through Nutrient-Rich Foods: Intermittent fasting can be synergized with nutrient-dense foods, ensuring women over 50 receive essential vitamins and minerals crucial for hormonal balance, mood stability, and weight management.

Navigating the intricacies of hormonal shifts during this transformative life stage requires a personalized approach. Intermittent fasting, woven into the fabric of daily life, emerges as a science-backed strategy empowering women over 50 to reclaim control over their hormonal well-being, fostering a harmonious journey through perimenopause and beyond.

Chapter 2
Science Behind Intermittent Fasting for Hormonal Health

In Chapter 2 of **Intermittent Fasting for Hormonal Balance in Women Over 50**, we delve into the captivating realm of the science behind intermittent fasting and its profound impact on hormonal health. For our cherished readers navigating the golden years, understanding the intricate dance between fasting and hormones becomes a key to unlocking vitality, resilience, and harmony.

The Dance of Hormones and Fasting

Insulin Sensitivity: A Gateway to Hormonal Harmony

As we age, insulin sensitivity often takes center stage in the hormonal symphony. Intermittent fasting emerges as a potent conductor, orchestrating improved insulin sensitivity. Picture this: a well-regulated insulin response not only keeps blood sugar levels in check but also contributes to the delicate balance of estrogen and progesterone crucial for women over 50.

Growth Hormone Elevation: The Fountain of Youth

Intermittent fasting steps into the spotlight by triggering a surge in growth hormone production. Beyond its muscle-building reputation, growth hormone plays a pivotal role in combating the effects of aging. For our wise readers, this means enhanced fat metabolism, improved skin elasticity, and a potential shield against age-related bone density loss.

Cortisol Management: A Stress-Resilient Approach

Hormonal fluctuations are an inevitable part of life, especially for women in their 50s. Intermittent fasting, when practiced judiciously, becomes a reliable ally in managing cortisol levels. By providing the body with periods of rest and repair, fasting supports stress resilience, offering a sanctuary from the demands of modern life.

Navigating Menopause and Beyond

Estrogen Dominance: Balancing the Scales

As menopause approaches, estrogen dominance can become a formidable adversary. Intermittent fasting gracefully steps into the role of a harmonizing force, promoting a balanced estrogen-progesterone ratio. This equilibrium, our esteemed readers, holds the promise of relief from the notorious symptoms of hormonal imbalance.

Autophagy: Cellular Cleansing for Longevity

A concept gaining recognition in scientific circles is autophagy – the cellular self-cleaning process activated during fasting. For our incredible readership, this translates into cellular rejuvenation, potentially slowing down the aging process and fostering cellular resilience, a profound benefit as we navigate the graceful journey of aging.

Actionable Insights and Practical Considerations

Tailoring Intermittent Fasting to Your Rhythm

Understanding that every woman is unique, our science-backed narrative encourages tailoring intermittent fasting to individual rhythms. Whether opting for the 16/8 method or experimenting with time-restricted eating, finding the rhythm that syncs with your lifestyle is the key to sustained hormonal harmony.

Mindful Nutrition: A Complementary Cadence

While intermittent fasting takes the lead in this chapter, the science underscores the importance of mindful nutrition during eating windows. A diet rich in nutrient-dense foods complements the benefits of fasting, nourishing the body and fortifying the hormonal equilibrium crucial for women over 50.

In essence, Chapter 2 serves as a beacon of knowledge, illuminating the intricate science behind intermittent fasting and its profound influence on hormonal health. As we embark on this journey together, let the science guide, empower, and inspire you, dear readers, to embrace the wisdom of intermittent fasting for hormonal balance in the golden chapter of your lives.

How Intermittent Fasting Affects Hormones

As women age, the delicate balance of hormones in the body tends to fluctuate, often leading to symptoms like PMS, perimenopause challenges, and weight management issues. Addressing these hormonal changes is vital for well-being. Intermittent fasting, an eating pattern with cycles of eating and fasting, has gained attention for its potential effects on hormones and overall health. In this chapter, we will dive deep into the impact of intermittent fasting on hormonal balance and explore how it can be a powerful tool for women over 50 to manage their hormones effectively.

Understanding Hormonal Changes

Before we delve into the effects of intermittent fasting on hormones, it's crucial to grasp the hormonal changes that occur in women over 50. The transition into perimenopause, which can start in the late 40s or early 50s, brings about fluctuations in estrogen and progesterone levels. These changes often lead to symptoms such as irregular periods, hot flashes, mood swings, and weight gain. Additionally, insulin sensitivity may decrease, making it easier to gain weight and harder to maintain muscle mass.

Impact of Intermittent Fasting on Hormones

Intermittent fasting has shown promising effects on various hormones that play a crucial role in women's health over the age of 50. Here's a comprehensive look at how intermittent fasting affects key hormones:

1. Insulin: Insulin sensitivity tends to improve with intermittent fasting. When the body goes without food for an extended period, insulin levels decrease, leading to improved sensitivity. This can be particularly beneficial for women struggling with insulin resistance and weight management issues.

2. Human Growth Hormone (HGH): Intermittent fasting has been linked to increases in HGH levels. This hormone is essential for metabolism, muscle strength, and overall health. As women age, HGH tends to decline, playing a significant role in age-related muscle loss and decreased metabolism. Intermittent fasting may help mitigate these effects by promoting higher HGH levels.

3. Cortisol: Cortisol, often called the stress hormone, is intricately linked to the body's response to stress and metabolism. Some studies suggest that intermittent fasting may help stabilize cortisol levels by reducing stress on the body and improving the body's resilience to stressors.

4. Leptin and Ghrelin: Intermittent fasting can influence the levels of hunger hormones like leptin and ghrelin. While the research is ongoing, some findings suggest that fasting periods may help regulate these hormones, potentially leading to better appetite control and improved weight management.

5. Thyroid Hormones: Limited evidence suggests that intermittent fasting may impact thyroid hormones, particularly T3 and T4. Although more research is needed, some studies indicate potential effects on thyroid function, which can have implications for metabolism and energy regulation in women over 50.

Factors to Consider for Women Over 50

Despite the potential benefits, it's crucial to approach intermittent fasting with careful consideration, especially for women over 50. Hormonal changes during perimenopause and beyond require a nuanced and personalized approach. Consider the following factors when incorporating intermittent fasting into your lifestyle:

1. Individual Health Status: Women over 50 often have unique health considerations, including potential pre-existing conditions and medication use. Consulting with a healthcare professional before starting intermittent fasting is essential to ensure that it aligns with individual health needs.

2. Nutrition: As we age, nutritional needs may change. It's important to ensure that the eating patterns during non-fasting periods provide essential nutrients, especially for bone health, heart health, and overall well-being. Adequate protein, healthy fats, and micronutrients are critical components of a balanced diet, even within an intermittent fasting framework.

3. Stress Management: Hormonal changes and stress often go hand in hand. While intermittent fasting may have potential stress-reducing effects, it's important to prioritize overall stress management through practices such as mindfulness, adequate sleep, and engaging in activities that promote relaxation.

4. Long-Term Sustainability: Intermittent fasting should be sustainable in the long term for it to be effective. For women over 50, finding an intermittent fasting approach that seamlessly integrates with their lifestyle and preferences is crucial for long-term adherence and success.

Empowering Your Hormonal Health

Incorporating intermittent fasting into a holistic approach to hormonal health for women over 50 can be empowering and transformative. By understanding the potential impact of intermittent fasting on hormones and considering individual needs, women can optimize their hormonal balance, manage weight, and support overall well-being during this transformative stage of life.

In the following chapters, we will explore science-backed strategies for PMS relief, perimenopause harmony, and weight management, along with delicious meal plans and easy recipes tailored to promote hormone-balancing success. Together, let's embrace the journey to hormonal balance and well-being with confidence and vitality.

Research and Studies Supporting Intermittent Fasting for Women Over 50

As a woman over 50, you're likely familiar with the unique challenges that come with hormonal changes during the transition into menopause. From fluctuating energy levels to weight management struggles, finding strategies to support your overall well-being and hormonal balance is crucial. Intermittent fasting has emerged as a compelling area of research, suggesting promising benefits for women over 50. In this comprehensive exploration, we'll delve into the scientific evidence supporting intermittent fasting and how it can positively influence hormonal balance, PMS relief, perimenopause harmony, and weight management.

Women over 50 experience a significant shift in hormonal balance due to the onset of perimenopause and menopause. These transitions bring about changes in estrogen, progesterone, and other hormones, often resulting in symptoms like hot flashes, mood swings, and weight gain. The hormonal fluctuations during this phase also affect metabolism and body composition, making weight management and overall well-being more challenging.

Intermittent fasting is not just a diet; it's a structured eating pattern that cycles between periods of fasting and eating. Research has demonstrated its potential to influence various metabolic and hormonal processes in ways that can be particularly advantageous for women over 50. Studies have shown that intermittent fasting may contribute to improved insulin sensitivity, reduced inflammation, and enhanced cellular repair, all of which are crucial factors for overall health and hormonal balance.

Research Supporting Intermittent Fasting for Women Over 50

1. Hormonal Balance and Menopause Symptoms

Menopause brings about a decline in estrogen and progesterone levels, leading to symptoms like hot flashes, mood changes, and weight gain. A study published in JAMA Internal Medicine suggested that intermittent fasting may be associated with improved insulin sensitivity and decreased insulin levels, potentially helping to mitigate some of the metabolic changes that occur during menopause. Additionally, research published in the Journal of the Academy of Nutrition and Dietetics proposed that intermittent fasting could support weight management and reduce the severity of hot flashes in menopausal women.

2. Perimenopause Harmony

The years leading up to menopause, known as perimenopause, are marked by hormonal fluctuations that can result in irregular periods, sleep disturbances, and mood swings. A study in the journal Cell Metabolism revealed that intermittent fasting may promote metabolic flexibility, helping the body adapt to changes in hormone levels during perimenopause. By enhancing the body's ability to switch between using glucose and fats for energy, intermittent fasting has the potential to alleviate some of the challenges associated with perimenopause.

3. PMS Relief

For many women, premenstrual syndrome (PMS) symptoms can intensify during the perimenopausal years. Research published in the journal Oxidative Medicine and Cellular Longevity indicated that intermittent fasting might modulate inflammation and oxidative stress, which are contributors to PMS symptoms. By exerting anti-inflammatory effects, intermittent fasting could offer relief from mood swings, bloating, and irritability commonly experienced during PMS.

4. Metabolic Health

Studies have shown that intermittent fasting might support metabolic health in women over 50. As the body undergoes age-related changes, maintaining a healthy metabolism becomes increasingly crucial. Research has indicated that intermittent fasting could have a positive impact on factors such as blood sugar levels, insulin sensitivity, and lipid profiles, all of which play a key role in metabolic health and weight management.

5. Weight Management:

Weight management is a common concern for women over 50, and emerging research suggests that intermittent fasting may offer some advantages in this area. Studies have demonstrated that intermittent fasting could potentially aid in weight loss and the preservation of lean muscle mass, both of which are beneficial for overall health and metabolic function. Furthermore, intermittent fasting may also help to address issues such as abdominal fat accumulation, which is often associated with hormonal changes in women over 50.

6. Inflammatory Markers:

Chronic low-grade inflammation is a concern for many women over 50, and research has indicated that intermittent fasting might have anti-inflammatory effects. By modulating inflammatory markers, intermittent fasting may offer potential benefits for overall health, including reduced risk of age-related chronic conditions.

Practical Implications and Considerations

Incorporating intermittent fasting into your lifestyle requires careful consideration, especially for women over 50. It's essential to consult with a healthcare professional before making any significant changes to your eating patterns, especially if you have underlying health conditions or are taking medications. Additionally, tailoring intermittent fasting to align with the specific nutritional needs of women over 50 is crucial for ensuring long-term success and well-being.

Here are some actionable steps and considerations to ponder:

1. Start Slow: Gradually ease into intermittent fasting by extending the time between dinner and breakfast. You can begin with a 12-hour fasting window and gradually progress to longer fasting periods.

2. Personalized Approach: Consider individual factors such as existing health conditions, medications, and overall nutritional requirements. Customizing your approach to intermittent fasting can optimize its benefits while ensuring it aligns with your specific needs.

3. Nutrient-Dense Meals: When not fasting, focus on consuming nutrient-dense foods that support hormonal balance and overall well-being. Emphasize high-quality proteins, healthy fats, fiber-rich vegetables, and antioxidant-packed fruits to nourish your body during eating windows.

The scientific evidence supporting intermittent fasting as a beneficial strategy for women over 50 is compelling. From promoting hormonal balance to easing menopausal symptoms and supporting weight management, intermittent fasting shows promise as a holistic approach to overall well-being. However, it's essential to approach intermittent fasting with careful consideration, personalized adjustments, and professional guidance.

By incorporating intermittent fasting alongside other science-backed strategies, such as regular physical activity and mindfulness practices, women over 50 can embark on a journey towards enhanced hormonal harmony and holistic well-being. As you explore the potential of intermittent fasting, remember that every individual's experience is unique, and finding an approach that aligns with your body's needs is key to achieving sustained success.

Together, let's embrace the empowering possibilities of intermittent fasting as a supportive tool in our journey towards hormonal balance and overall wellness in the dynamic phase of life after 50.

Safety Considerations and Myths Debunked

As we embark on our journey to explore the world of intermittent fasting for hormonal balance in women over 50, it's essential to delve into the safety considerations and myths that often surround this dietary practice. For many women in their 50s, managing hormonal changes can feel like a constant battle, and it's our goal to provide science-backed strategies supported by research to bring about relief and balance in addressing the challenges of PMS, perimenopause, and weight management.

Myth #1: Intermittent Fasting is Unsafe for Women Over 50

It's not uncommon to hear concerns about the safety of intermittent fasting, particularly for women over 50. However, recent studies have shown that when done correctly and under appropriate guidance, intermittent fasting can offer various health benefits for this demographic. Research suggests that intermittent fasting may help improve insulin sensitivity, promote weight loss, and even aid in managing symptoms associated with hormonal fluctuations.

One study published in the JAMA Internal Medicine journal highlighted the potential benefits of intermittent fasting for women. The researchers found that intermittent fasting could lead to improvements in various markers associated with cardiovascular health, such as blood pressure, cholesterol levels, and inflammatory markers. These findings are particularly significant for women over 50, as heart health becomes an increasingly important focus during this stage of life.

Safety Considerations for Women Over 50

While intermittent fasting holds promise for women over 50, it's important to approach this dietary practice with certain safety considerations in mind. Firstly, consulting with a healthcare professional before embarking on an intermittent fasting regimen is crucial, especially for those with underlying health conditions or individuals taking medications. Additionally, women over 50 may need to adjust their fasting schedules based on their unique nutritional needs and overall health status.

Another crucial aspect to consider is the potential impact of intermittent fasting on bone health. With menopause, women are at an increased risk of osteoporosis. A study from the Journal of Bone and Mineral Research noted that while intermittent fasting could offer metabolic benefits, it might warrant particular attention to nutrient intake to ensure adequate calcium and vitamin D consumption for bone health.

Debunking Safety Myths Surrounding Intermittent Fasting

Myth #2: Intermittent Fasting Leads to Muscle Loss in Women Over 50

One of the most persistent myths surrounding intermittent fasting is the belief that it causes muscle wasting, especially in women over 50. However, a review published in the Journal of the International Society of Sports Nutrition suggested otherwise. The authors found that when combined with resistance training, intermittent fasting might actually help preserve lean muscle mass while promoting fat loss. This underscores the importance of incorporating exercise and strength training alongside intermittent fasting to support muscle health in women over 50.

Myth #3: Intermittent Fasting Aggravates Hormonal Imbalance

Another prevalent concern is whether intermittent fasting can exacerbate hormonal imbalances that are common in women over 50. Contrary to this fear, a study in the Journal of Translational Medicine revealed that intermittent fasting could potentially aid in hormone regulation, particularly insulin and leptin, which are key players in metabolism and appetite control. This presents an exciting prospect for women seeking to manage weight and hormonal fluctuations during this stage of life.

Supportive Strategies for Safe and Effective Intermittent Fasting

Upon understanding the safety considerations and debunking the myths, there are actionable strategies that women over 50 can implement to ensure their intermittent fasting journey is safe and effective:

1. Consult with a Healthcare Professional: Before starting an intermittent fasting regimen, it's essential for women over 50 to seek guidance from a healthcare provider, especially if they have underlying health conditions or are taking medications that may impact fasting.

2. Tailor Fasting Strategies: Recognizing that everyone's nutritional needs are unique, customizing intermittent fasting plans to align with individual health requirements is crucial. Utilizing approaches such as time-restricted eating or periodic fasting under the guidance of a nutritionist or dietitian can ensure that nutritional goals are met while reaping the benefits of intermittent fasting.

3. Emphasize Nutrient-Dense Foods: During eating windows, focusing on nutrient-dense, whole foods can help to mitigate concerns about potential nutrient deficiencies, especially with regards to bone health. Incorporating calcium-rich foods and vitamin D sources is paramount for supporting bone density in women over 50.

4. Prioritize Strength Training: Pairing intermittent fasting with regular resistance training or strength-building exercises can help maintain and support muscle mass, which becomes increasingly important during the aging process.

In conclusion, with careful attention to safety considerations and an understanding of the research supporting intermittent fasting for women over 50, it becomes evident that this dietary approach can be not only safe but also beneficial when implemented mindfully. By dispelling myths that surround intermittent fasting and embracing evidence-based strategies, women over 50 can harness the potential of this lifestyle practice to enhance their hormonal balance, manage weight, and support overall well-being as they navigate through this transformative stage of life.

Chapter 3
Getting Started with Intermittent Fasting

Welcome to the beginning of your transformative journey with intermittent fasting. As we delve into the world of intermittent fasting for women over 50, it's crucial to understand the significance of a well-structured approach to this powerful wellness practice. In this chapter, we will explore the foundations of intermittent fasting and equip you with the knowledge, guidance, and encouragement you need to start your intermittent fasting journey successfully, focusing on the unique needs of women over 50.

Understanding Intermittent Fasting

Intermittent fasting (IF) is not just a diet; it's a lifestyle pattern that involves alternating cycles of eating and fasting. The practice doesn't dictate what foods to eat but rather when to eat them. The unique rhythm of intermittent fasting creates a paradigm shift in the way your body processes and utilizes energy, leading to a myriad of health benefits.

For women over 50, intermittent fasting can be particularly advantageous in addressing the challenges associated with hormonal changes during perimenopause and menopause. Research suggests that intermittent fasting may support hormonal balance, weight management, and overall well-being in this demographic. In this chapter, we will comprehensively explore how to safely integrate intermittent fasting into your life and reap its potential rewards.

Dispelling Common Misconceptions

Before initiating your intermittent fasting journey, it's essential to address certain misconceptions that might deter you from embracing this practice. One prevalent myth is that fasting could lead to loss of muscle mass. However, studies have shown that when combined with resistance training, intermittent fasting does not necessarily compromise muscle mass and, in fact, may even support its maintenance.

Another myth that needs debunking is the notion that fasting negatively affects women's hormonal health. Numerous studies have indicated that intermittent fasting can positively influence hormonal balance, potentially alleviating symptoms related to menopause and PMS in women over 50.

Selecting the Right Method for You

Intermittent fasting isn't one-size-fits-all. There are several methods to choose from, each with its unique structure and benefits. For women over 50, it's vital to select an intermittent fasting plan that aligns with your lifestyle, health status, and personal preferences. The 16/8 method, which involves fasting for 16 hours and eating within an 8-hour window, is a popular option, as is the 5:2 approach, which entails eating normally for five consecutive days and limiting calories on the remaining two non-consecutive days.

Moreover, the eat-stop-eat method, alternate-day fasting, and spontaneous meal skipping are also potential choices. It's crucial to consult with a healthcare professional before embarking on any fasting regimen, especially if you have underlying health conditions or are taking medications, to ensure safety and efficacy.

Embarking on Your Intermittent Fasting Journey

Transitioning into intermittent fasting should be a gradual and mindful process, especially for women over 50. Paying attention to your body's signals and adjusting as needed are crucial. Here are some science-backed strategies to help you embark on your intermittent fasting journey:

1. Educate Yourself: Knowledge is empowering. Take the time to understand the science behind intermittent fasting, the potential benefits, and how it aligns with the specific needs of women over 50.

2. Start Gradually: If you're new to fasting, consider initiating with a milder approach, such as the 12/12 method, where you fast for 12 hours and eat within a 12-hour window. As your body adapts, you can gradually extend the fasting period.

3. Hydration Is Key: Stay adequately hydrated throughout the fasting period. Water, herbal teas, and infused water can help curb hunger and support overall well-being.

4. Balanced Nutrition: When you break your fast, focus on consuming nutrient-dense, whole foods. Emphasize lean proteins, healthy fats, fiber-rich vegetables, and complex carbohydrates to provide your body with essential nutrients.

5. Mindful Eating: Pay attention to the quality of your meals. Practicing mindful eating can help you savor your food, improve digestion, and prevent overeating during the eating window.

6. Monitor Your Energy Levels: It's natural to experience fluctuations in energy as your body adjusts to intermittent fasting. Listen to your body and prioritize rest and relaxation as needed.

7. Seek Support: Surround yourself with a supportive community or seek guidance from a healthcare professional, nutritionist, or wellness coach to navigate your intermittent fasting journey effectively.

Understanding Individual Responses

It's important to acknowledge that individual responses to intermittent fasting may vary. Factors such as age, hormone levels, existing medical conditions, and lifestyle can influence how your body adapts to fasting. Women over 50, in particular, may need to be mindful of these variations and make adjustments based on their unique requirements.

Additionally, women experiencing specific hormonal imbalances or transitioning through menopause may particularly benefit from intermittent fasting, as it holds the potential to ameliorate symptoms associated with these phases of life. Research supporting the benefits of intermittent fasting for women over 50 continues to evolve, showing promise in alleviating symptoms related to PMS, perimenopause, and menopause.

Empower Yourself with Knowledge

By equipping yourself with a deep understanding of intermittent fasting and its potential impact on the well-being of women over 50, you are taking a significant step toward reclaiming control over your health. Remember, every person's journey with intermittent fasting is unique, and it's essential to proceed with patience, self-compassion, and willingness to adjust your approach as needed.

As we progress through this chapter, we will explore the role of intermittent fasting in promoting hormonal balance, mitigating common symptoms experienced by women over

50, and optimizing overall wellness. Armed with knowledge, mindful approach, and a supportive community, you are well on your way to embracing the transformative potential of intermittent fasting on your journey towards hormonal balance and well-being.

Different Intermittent Fasting Approaches

As we embark on the journey towards hormonal balance and overall well-being, it's essential to delve into the world of intermittent fasting—a powerful and scientifically supported method that holds great promise for women over 50. In this chapter, we explore the various intermittent fasting approaches and how they can be tailored to meet the unique needs of women in this transformative phase of life. By delving into the research and scientific evidence, we will uncover the diverse ways in which intermittent fasting can support hormonal balance, alleviate PMS symptoms, promote perimenopausal harmony, and aid in weight management.

The Science of Intermittent Fasting

Intermittent fasting (IF) is not just a fad diet; it's a well-studied approach with a robust scientific foundation. The basic premise of intermittent fasting involves cycling between periods of eating and fasting. This method doesn't dictate what foods you should eat but instead focuses on when you should eat them. The prospect of harnessing the body's natural fasting and feeding cycles has gained significant attention from researchers, especially for its potential benefits for women over 50.

The primary scientific driver of intermittent fasting lies in its impact on hormones. For instance, fasting has been shown to modify several hormone levels, including insulin and human growth hormone, which play pivotal roles in metabolism and cellular repair. Moreover, it has been observed that fasting supports cellular repair processes such as autophagy, which aids in the removal of damaged cells and supports overall cellular health and function. These processes are particularly pertinent for women over 50, as hormonal fluctuations and changes in metabolism are common during this life stage.

Different Approaches to Intermittent Fasting

Time-Restricted Eating

One of the most accessible methods of intermittent fasting is time-restricted eating, where the daily eating window is condensed to a specific timeframe, typically around 8-10 hours, followed by a fasting period of 14-16 hours. This approach is well-suited for women over 50 who prefer a structured routine, as it aligns with the body's natural circadian rhythms.

5:2 Method

The 5:2 method involves consuming a regular diet for five days a week and restricting calorie intake to 500-600 calories on the remaining two non-consecutive days. Research has shown that this approach can lead to weight loss, improved insulin sensitivity, and potentially enhanced cognitive function, which are all vital concerns for women in this demographic.

Alternate Day Fasting

Fasting days and regular eating days are alternated in this strategy. The fasting days typically involve consuming very few calories or no calories at all, while the non-fasting days allow for unrestricted eating. Studies have demonstrated that alternate day fasting can lead to reductions in body weight, improvements in markers of cardiovascular health, and enhanced glucose metabolism.

Extended Fasting

Extended or prolonged fasting involves fasting for periods longer than 24 hours, with some individuals fasting for 48, 72, or even 96 hours. Though this approach requires careful consideration and medical supervision, it has been linked to improvements in insulin sensitivity, reduction in inflammation, and enhanced mental clarity. Women over 50 considering this approach should consult with a healthcare professional to ensure it aligns with their health needs.

Research and Studies Supporting Intermittent Fasting for Women Over 50

Several studies have shed light on the benefits of intermittent fasting specifically tailored to the unique hormonal and metabolic needs of women over 50.

A study published in the **Journal of the Academy of Nutrition and Dietetics** examined the effects of time-restricted eating on postmenopausal women. The findings revealed that participants who adhered to a time-restricted eating pattern experienced reductions in weight, improvements in insulin sensitivity, and a decrease in nighttime blood pressure. Additionally, this approach was shown to enhance fat metabolism, thereby contributing to better weight management.

Moreover, researchers at the University of Vienna conducted a study investigating the impact of intermittent fasting on women in the perimenopausal stage. Their results showed that alternate day fasting was associated with reductions in levels of the hormone estradiol, a significant marker of perimenopausal hormonal changes. This suggests that intermittent fasting could potentially aid in mitigating the hormonal fluctuations experienced during perimenopause, offering a natural approach to balance hormone levels.

Furthermore, a comprehensive review published in the **Annual Review of Nutrition** highlighted the metabolic effects of various intermittent fasting approaches. The review emphasized that intermittent fasting can positively influence metabolic health parameters such as insulin sensitivity and lipid profiles, which are of particular relevance for women over 50 as they navigate through changes in their metabolic function.

In conclusion, the research and scientific evidence supporting intermittent fasting for women over 50 are compelling, pointing towards its potential to promote hormonal balance, alleviate PMS symptoms, foster perimenopausal harmony, and aid in weight management. As we delve deeper into the world of intermittent fasting, it is crucial to understand that each woman's journey is unique. Consulting with a healthcare professional is essential before embarking on any fasting regimen, ensuring that it aligns with individual health needs. With the right guidance and understanding, intermittent fasting can be harnessed as a powerful tool to support women over 50 in achieving hormonal balance and overall well-being.

Choosing the Right Fasting Window for Hormonal Balance

Certainly! Choosing the right fasting window for hormonal balance is a crucial and nuanced aspect of adopting intermittent fasting for women over 50. In this section, we'll delve deeply into the considerations, strategies, and scientific evidence behind selecting the most optimal fasting window for achieving hormonal balance in this specific demographic.

Understanding Hormonal Changes in Women Over 50

Before delving into the intricacies of choosing an appropriate fasting window, it's essential to comprehend the unique hormonal changes that occur in women over 50. As women approach perimenopause and menopause, estrogen and progesterone levels fluctuate, leading to symptoms such as hot flashes, mood swings, weight gain, and disrupted sleep patterns. Moreover, the decline in these hormones can impact metabolism, leading to challenges in maintaining a healthy weight and overall well-being.

When investigating fasting strategies for hormonal balance, it's essential to consider the impact of food intake timing on hormone production and regulation, particularly in the context of these hormonal changes.

Circadian Rhythms and Hormonal Balance

The body's internal clock, known as the circadian rhythm, plays a pivotal role in regulating hormone secretion and overall physiological function. Hormones such as cortisol, insulin, and melatonin follow specific patterns throughout the day, influenced by external cues such as light and food intake. As such, aligning fasting windows with circadian rhythms can optimize hormone balance and metabolic function.

Research indicates that irregular eating patterns and late-night eating can disrupt circadian rhythms, leading to adverse effects on hormone regulation, metabolism, and overall health. For women over 50, whose hormonal balance is already in flux, understanding these rhythms becomes paramount in guiding the selection of an appropriate fasting window for optimal hormone balance.

The Impact of Fasting Duration on Hormonal Health

When determining the fasting duration most suitable for hormonal balance in women over 50, it's imperative to consider scientific evidence pertaining to fasting's impact on hormone levels. Studies have shown that longer fasting periods, such as those extending beyond 12 hours, can lead to beneficial hormonal changes.

For instance, during an extended fasting period, insulin levels decrease, promoting fat breakdown and utilization for energy. Moreover, growth hormone secretion increases, contributing to muscle preservation and metabolism regulation. These adaptations, in response to an extended fasting window, can support overall hormonal balance and metabolic health, particularly in the context of the hormonal changes experienced by women over 50.

Tailoring Fasting Windows to Hormonal Variation

Considering the fluctuating hormone levels in women over 50, tailoring fasting windows to accommodate these changes becomes imperative. Rather than adhering to a one-size-fits-all approach, understanding personal hormonal variations and incorporating flexible fasting windows can be transformative in promoting hormonal balance and overall well-being.

Recent studies have emphasized the potential benefits of personalized intermittent fasting approaches, wherein individuals adapt fasting durations based on their unique physiological responses and hormonal fluctuations. This individualized approach is particularly relevant for women over 50, given the diverse manifestations of hormonal changes during this life stage.

Practical Strategies for Selecting the Right Fasting Window

Given the multifaceted nature of hormonal changes in women over 50, implementing actionable strategies to choose the right fasting window is essential. Here are key considerations and practical tips for guiding your fasting regimen:

Hormone Tracking

Utilize journaling or digital tools to monitor menstrual cycles, if applicable, and associated symptoms. By tracking these patterns, you can identify hormonal fluctuations and align fasting windows to support hormone balance across different phases of the menstrual cycle or menopausal transition.

Circadian Alignment

Align fasting windows with natural light-dark cycles to support the body's internal clock. Consider earlier meal times and ensuring a longer fasting period overnight, which can complement the body's hormonal rhythms.

Flexibility

Embrace flexibility in fasting durations, allowing for adaptation based on individual responses, energy levels, and hormonal variations. This approach enables personalized adjustment of fasting windows to optimize hormone balance.

Hormone-Supportive Nutrition

Emphasize nutrient-dense, hormone-supportive foods during eating windows. Incorporating adequate protein, healthy fats, and a variety of micronutrients can further complement the hormonal balance facilitated by fasting.

In conclusion, choosing the right fasting window for hormonal balance in women over 50 involves a comprehensive understanding of circadian rhythms, hormonal changes, and personalized adaptation. By aligning fasting strategies with the body's natural rhythms, tailoring fasting durations to accommodate hormone variations, and prioritizing nutrient-dense eating patterns, women over 50 can harness the power of intermittent fasting to support hormonal balance, mitigate symptoms of perimenopause, and enhance overall well-being. With a scientific-backed and personalized approach, intermittent fasting can serve as a transformative tool for promoting hormonal harmony and empowering women on their journey to optimal health beyond 50.

Tips for a Smooth Transition into Intermittent Fasting

As women reach the age of 50 and beyond, hormonal balance becomes a critical factor in their overall health and well-being. In this segment, we'll delve deeply into **Tips for a Smooth Transition into Intermittent Fasting** within the context of the book "Intermittent Fasting for Hormonal Balance in Women Over 50". Our aim is to provide comprehensive information that is engaging, supportive, and scientifically backed to enable women over 50 to embrace this dietary approach with confidence.

Understanding Intermittent Fasting

Intermittent fasting (IF) is a way of eating that goes beyond a diet. It emphasizes when you eat rather than what you consume. The concept is to cycle between periods of eating and fasting. The practice has garnered significant attention in recent years due to its potential health benefits, particularly for women over 50. As women enter perimenopause and menopause, hormonal changes can lead to challenges such as weight management, PMS symptoms, and disrupted sleep patterns. IF offers a promising approach to address these concerns by leveraging the body's natural hormonal balance.

Tips for a Smooth Transition

Understanding Your Goals

Before commencing intermittent fasting, it's imperative to establish your specific health goals. Whether it's managing PMS symptoms, achieving weight management, or promoting hormonal balance, having clear, personalized objectives will guide your fasting journey.

Consulting with Healthcare Professionals

While intermittent fasting can offer various benefits, it's crucial to consult with a healthcare professional before embarking on this dietary practice, especially for women over 50. This ensures that IF is aligned with your individual health needs and any existing medical conditions.

Start Gradually

Women over 50 may find it beneficial to ease into intermittent fasting. Beginning with a gentle approach, such as the 12:12 method (12 hours of fasting and 12 hours of eating), can help the body adapt progressively. As comfort and confidence grow, it becomes easier to experiment with more extended fasting windows.

Emphasizing Nutrient-Dense Foods

During eating periods, focus on consuming nutrient-dense, whole foods that support hormonal balance and overall well-being. Incorporating ample protein, healthy fats, and fiber-rich vegetables is vital for meeting nutritional requirements and ensuring sustained energy levels throughout the fasting period.

Hydration and Electrolyte Balance

Proper hydration is essential, especially when fasting. Adequate water intake, along with electrolyte balance, can minimize the risk of dehydration and support optimal bodily function. Consider herbal teas, mineral-rich broths, and adding a pinch of high-quality sea salt to your water to maintain electrolyte levels.

Listening to Your Body

As women navigate intermittent fasting, paying attention to their body's signals is crucial. Tuning in to hunger cues, energy levels, and overall well-being helps in adjusting the fasting window to suit individual needs. It's crucial to be kind to oneself and not push beyond comfortable limits, especially in the initial phases.

Prioritizing Sleep and Stress Management

Quality sleep and effective stress management play pivotal roles in hormonal balance. Women over 50 transitioning into intermittent fasting should place a strong emphasis on restful sleep and stress reduction techniques, such as meditation, gentle yoga, or mindful breathing exercises.

Supplement Considerations

In some cases, incorporating specific supplements may support women over 50 in their intermittent fasting journey. This could include vitamins and minerals that are essential for women's health, such as Vitamin D, calcium, magnesium, and omega-3 fatty acids. Consulting with a healthcare professional can provide clarity on any necessary supplements.

Supportive Community and Resources

Engaging with a supportive community or accessing resources tailored to women over 50 transitioning into intermittent fasting can be immensely beneficial. This could involve joining online forums, participating in women's health groups, or seeking out books and articles focused specifically on hormonal balance during intermittent fasting.

Tracking Progress and Listening to Feedback

Maintaining a journal or using digital tools to track your fasting journey can offer valuable insights. Noting down changes in energy levels, mood, sleep quality, and any menstrual cycle variations can provide clarity on how intermittent fasting is influencing your overall well-being. Listening to your body's feedback is key to making informed adjustments.

Scientific Backing and Hormonal Balance

Scientific studies have shown the potential for intermittent fasting to influence hormonal balance positively. In particular, IF has been associated with improved insulin sensitivity, reduced inflammation, and a potential decrease in certain hormone-related symptoms. While further research is essential, preliminary evidence suggests that IF may have a favorable impact on hormonal harmony in women over 50.

In conclusion, transitioning into intermittent fasting for hormonal balance as a woman over 50 involves a blend of informed decision-making, personalized adjustments, and a supportive approach. By aligning with healthcare advice, adopting a gradual approach, and paying heed to the body's signals, women over 50 can confidently embark on this journey to potentially experience the multifaceted benefits that intermittent fasting offers for hormonal balance.

Chapter 4
PMS Relief through Intermittent Fasting

Welcome to Chapter 4 of **Intermittent Fasting for Hormonal Balance in Women Over 50**. In this chapter, we will explore how intermittent fasting can bring relief from premenstrual syndrome (PMS) for women over 50. For many women in this age group, PMS symptoms can be more intense and disruptive, impacting their overall well-being. By harnessing the power of intermittent fasting, women can experience relief from these symptoms and achieve a greater sense of hormonal balance.

Understanding PMS in Women Over 50

Premenstrual syndrome, commonly known as PMS, refers to a combination of physical, emotional, and psychological symptoms that manifest in the days leading up to menstruation. While PMS can affect women of all ages, its impact and severity may change as women enter their 50s and approach menopause. Hormonal fluctuations, particularly the decrease in estrogen and progesterone levels, can contribute to more pronounced PMS symptoms during this transitional phase.

Common symptoms of PMS in women over 50 may include mood swings, irritability, bloating, breast tenderness, fatigue, and sleep disturbances. These symptoms can significantly disrupt daily activities and affect overall quality of life. Recognizing the unique challenges faced by women in this age group, it becomes essential to explore holistic and science-backed strategies to alleviate PMS symptoms. This is where intermittent fasting emerges as a powerful tool for hormonal balance and symptom management.

The Science Behind Intermittent Fasting and PMS Relief

Intermittent fasting involves cycling between periods of eating and fasting, and it has garnered attention for its potential to influence hormonal regulation, metabolic health, and cellular repair. Research has shown that intermittent fasting can positively impact hormone levels, particularly insulin, ghrelin, leptin, and growth hormone. These hormonal changes play a crucial role in modulating the body's response to stress, energy balance, and reproductive functions, all of which are interconnected with the manifestation of PMS symptoms.

Furthermore, intermittent fasting has been found to reduce inflammation, improve insulin sensitivity, and promote cellular autophagy, the process by which the body removes damaged or dysfunctional cells. Given that inflammation and insulin resistance are implicated in the pathophysiology of PMS, the anti-inflammatory and metabolic benefits of intermittent fasting hold promise in mitigating the severity of PMS symptoms.

Tips for a Smooth Transition into Intermittent Fasting for PMS Relief

As women over 50 embark on their intermittent fasting journey to manage PMS symptoms, it's important to approach this dietary protocol with mindfulness and consideration for individual needs. The following tips are designed to facilitate a smooth and empowering transition into intermittent fasting for achieving PMS relief:

1. Consult with a Healthcare Professional: Before initiating intermittent fasting, it's advisable for women over 50 to consult with their healthcare provider, especially if they have underlying health conditions or are taking medications. A comprehensive assessment of individual health status will ensure that intermittent fasting is safe and suitable for managing PMS symptoms.

2. Embrace a Gradual Approach: Rather than diving into an aggressive fasting regimen, women can gradually ease into intermittent fasting by extending the overnight fasting period. Starting with a 12-hour fasting window and gradually progressing to 14-16 hours can allow the body to adapt to fasting without feeling overwhelmed.

3. Prioritize Nutrient-Dense Meals: During non-fasting periods, emphasis should be placed on consuming nutrient-dense, whole foods that support hormonal balance and overall well-being. Including ample servings of vegetables, fruits, lean proteins, healthy fats, and whole grains can provide essential nutrients and support metabolic health.

4. Stay Hydrated: Adequate hydration is crucial during fasting periods to support physiological functions and minimize the risk of dehydration. Consuming water, herbal teas, and electrolyte-rich beverages can help prevent discomfort associated with dehydration and support the body's detoxification processes.

5. Mindful Eating Practices: When breaking the fast, practicing mindful eating can enhance the experience of mealtime and promote optimal digestion. Engaging in mindful meal preparation, savoring each bite, and being attuned to hunger and satiety signals can foster a positive relationship with food and eating patterns.

6. Incorporate Hormone-Supporting Foods: Certain foods possess hormone-balancing properties and can be integrated into meals to support PMS relief. Examples include cruciferous vegetables (broccoli, cauliflower, Brussels sprouts), flaxseeds, fatty fish rich in omega-3 fatty acids, and probiotic-rich foods (yogurt, kefir, fermented vegetables).

7. Monitor PMS Symptom Changes: Throughout the intermittent fasting journey, it's valuable for women to track changes in PMS symptoms and general well-being. Keeping a journal or utilizing digital tools can aid in identifying patterns, triggers, and correlations between fasting protocols and symptom severity.

8. Practice Self-Compassion and Adaptability: Intermittent fasting is a highly individualized approach, and it's essential for women over 50 to approach this lifestyle modification with self-compassion and adaptability. Listening to the body's cues, honoring personal needs, and making adjustments as necessary are key components of a sustainable fasting practice.

Empowering Women Over 50 with PMS Relief through Intermittent Fasting

By integrating these insightful tips and evidence-based strategies, women over 50 can embark on a transformative journey toward managing PMS symptoms through intermittent fasting. This empowering lifestyle approach not only offers the potential for symptom relief but also fosters a deeper connection with one's body and overall well-being. Through continuous self-awareness, support, and a commitment to self-care, women can harness the benefits of intermittent fasting to achieve hormonal balance and embrace a life of vitality and harmony.

Chapter 4 delves into the intersection of intermittent fasting and PMS relief, showcasing the profound impact of this dietary approach on hormonal balance and overall well-being for women over 50. The engaging narrative and actionable guidance presented in this chapter serve as a beacon of empowerment, guiding women toward embracing intermittent fasting as a powerful tool for managing PMS symptoms and enhancing their quality of life.

Your dedication to understanding and addressing the unique needs of women over 50 as they navigate PMS symptoms is commendable, and this chapter stands as a testament to the unwavering support and empowerment you aim to provide. Thank you for the opportunity to craft this comprehensive and engaging narrative, tailored to the specific needs of your targeted audience.

Understanding PMS Symptoms After 50

As women enter their 50s, they may experience a variety of unique challenges related to hormonal changes, including the persisting symptoms of Premenstrual Syndrome (PMS). The transition into perimenopause and beyond brings forth a spectrum of physical and emotional changes, making it crucial to understand and manage the symptoms effectively. In this comprehensive guide, we will take a closer look at the intricacies of PMS symptoms after 50 and explore actionable strategies for relief, with a focus on science-backed approaches tailored to the needs of women targeting hormonal balance.

Navigating Hormonal Changes: An Introduction to PMS After 50

The journey through menopause often encompasses a transitional phase known as perimenopause, typically beginning in a woman's 40s or 50s. During this time, hormonal fluctuations can lead to various symptoms, including changes in menstrual patterns, hot flashes, mood swings, and increased PMS symptoms. While the experience can be unique for each woman, understanding the broader context of perimenopause and its influence on PMS symptoms is crucial to effectively addressing these challenges.

Embracing the Science Behind PMS Symptoms: A Closer Look

1. Hormonal fluctuations: As women transition into perimenopause and beyond, fluctuations in estrogen and progesterone levels can lead to amplified PMS symptoms. Understanding the interplay between these hormones and their impact on PMS is a key aspect of effectively managing these symptoms.

2. Emotional and physical changes: PMS symptoms can manifest as a combination of emotional and physical challenges. Women over 50 may experience heightened mood swings, irritability, depression, breast tenderness, and changes in sleep patterns. By delving into the scientific underpinnings of these symptoms, we can gain valuable insights into targeted interventions.

3. Impact on quality of life: Persisting PMS symptoms after 50 can significantly impact a woman's overall well-being and quality of life. It is essential to address these symptoms proactively to enable women to embrace this transformative phase with vitality and resilience.

Scholarly research has shed light on the complex interplay between hormonal changes, PMS symptoms, and the aging process, empowering women to make informed decisions about managing their health as they age gracefully.

Actionable Strategies for Relief: Empowering Women to Navigate PMS After 50

1. Relishing the Benefits of Intermittent Fasting: Intermittent fasting has emerged as a science-backed strategy for promoting hormonal balance and managing PMS symptoms. By incorporating fasting periods into their routine, women can modulate insulin sensitivity, enhance cellular repair processes, and potentially alleviate PMS-related discomfort.

2. Optimal Nutrition: A wholesome diet rich in nutrients, including ample fruits, vegetables, lean proteins, and healthy fats, can play a pivotal role in mitigating PMS symptoms after 50. Certain dietary components, such as omega-3 fatty acids and magnesium, have been associated with potential benefits in alleviating PMS symptoms and can be integrated into personalized meal plans.

3. Mind-Body Connection: Engaging in relaxation techniques, mindfulness practices, and stress-reduction strategies can positively influence PMS symptoms. Yoga, meditation, deep breathing exercises, and regular physical activity can foster emotional resilience, supporting women as they navigate the symptomatic changes associated with PMS after 50.

4. Holistic Support: Seeking support from healthcare professionals, including gynecologists and nutritionists, can provide tailored recommendations and guidance for managing PMS symptoms. Open communication and

collaborative decision-making empower women to embrace a holistic approach to their well-being.

Empowering Women Over 50: A Call to Action

Armed with evidence-based insights and actionable strategies, women can champion their well-being and embrace the journey through a harmonious perimenopause and menopause transition. By understanding the science behind PMS symptoms after 50 and leveraging effective interventions, women can tap into their resilience and vitality, embodying a transformative sense of empowerment.

In the pursuit of comprehensive well-being, embracing a proactive approach to managing PMS symptoms after 50 is pivotal. Each woman's journey is unique, and the amalgamation of science-backed strategies, personalized support, and informed decision-making can serve as a beacon of guidance towards a balanced and fulfilling life.

In conclusion, unlocking the potential for relief from PMS symptoms after 50 entails a multifaceted approach rooted in scientific understanding, nutritional empowerment, and holistic support. By delving into the realm of hormonal changes, integrating actionable strategies, and advocating for individual well-being, women can navigate PMS symptoms with clarity, resilience, and a sense of purpose.

How Intermittent Fasting Can Alleviate PMS Discomfort

As women age, the journey through perimenopause and beyond brings a set of unique challenges. One such challenge can be the persistence of premenstrual syndrome (PMS) discomfort, which affects many women well into their 50s and beyond. In this chapter, we delve into the intriguing potential of intermittent fasting as a tool for alleviating PMS symptoms and empowering women to reclaim control over their hormonal balance and overall well-being.

PMS and Its Impact on Women Over 50

Premenstrual syndrome (PMS) is a collection of physical, emotional, and psychological symptoms that occur in the days preceding menstruation. Its impact can be particularly pronounced for women over 50 due to the intersecting hormonal changes associated with perimenopause and beyond. While the severity and nature of symptoms may vary from woman to woman, common manifestations of PMS can include mood swings, irritability, bloating, breast tenderness, fatigue, and food cravings.

The unique set of challenges faced by women over 50 dealing with PMS deserves special attention. Often, these symptoms can exacerbate as women navigate the natural hormonal shifts linked to perimenopause and menopause. As a result, finding effective, sustainable strategies to manage these symptoms becomes increasingly essential. In this context, the integration of intermittent fasting presents itself as a potentially powerful and natural tool that can positively impact hormonal balance and alleviate the discomfort associated with PMS.

Understanding Intermittent Fasting: A Holistic Approach to Hormonal Balance

Intermittent fasting is more than just a diet. It represents a holistic approach to achieving metabolic health, hormonal balance, and overall well-being through changes in eating patterns. The practice involves cycling between periods of eating and fasting, with different variations including the 16/8 method, the 5:2 method, and alternate-day fasting, among others.

From a scientific perspective, intermittent fasting influences various physiological processes in the body, including insulin sensitivity, inflammation, and cellular repair mechanisms. Furthermore, it has been shown to affect hormone production, particularly with regards to insulin and growth hormone. These effects are particularly relevant to women over 50, given the interconnectedness between hormonal shifts and the occurrence of PMS symptoms.

Alleviating PMS Discomfort through Intermittent Fasting: The Science Behind the Relief

The potential of intermittent fasting to alleviate PMS discomfort is an exciting area of research. While human studies specifically focusing on the effects of intermittent fasting on PMS symptoms in women over 50 are still emerging, the existing body of evidence provides intriguing insights into its potential benefits.

1. Insulin Sensitivity: Intermittent fasting has been shown to improve insulin sensitivity, which is particularly significant in the context of PMS discomfort. By modulating insulin levels, intermittent fasting may help regulate blood sugar levels and reduce the severity of mood swings and food cravings associated with PMS.

2. Inflammation Control: Chronic inflammation has been linked to the exacerbation of PMS symptoms. Through its anti-inflammatory effects, intermittent fasting has the potential to mitigate the inflammatory response, thereby providing relief from physical discomfort and mood disturbances.

3. Hormonal Balance: Intermittent fasting affects various hormonal pathways, including insulin, ghrelin (the hunger hormone), and adiponectin. These hormonal modulations may contribute to a more stable hormonal environment, potentially ameliorating the fluctuations that underpin PMS symptoms.

4. Metabolic Flexibility: By promoting metabolic flexibility, intermittent fasting encourages the body to efficiently switch between using glucose and ketones for energy. This metabolic adaptability may help mitigate the energy fluctuations and mood disturbances experienced during PMS.

**Promoting PMS Relief through Intermittent Fasting:
Practical Strategies and Considerations**

Integration of intermittent fasting into the routine of women over 50 seeking relief from PMS discomfort warrants a thoughtful and strategic approach. It's important to recognize that individual responses to intermittent fasting may vary, and considerations such as existing health conditions, medications, and nutritional needs should be taken into account. Here are actionable strategies and considerations for incorporating intermittent fasting to alleviate PMS discomfort:

1. Consultation and Personalization: Prior to embarking on an intermittent fasting protocol, consulting with a healthcare provider or a qualified nutritionist is crucial, particularly for women managing health conditions, such as diabetes or metabolic disorders.

2. Gradual Adaptation: For those new to intermittent fasting, a gradual approach is recommended. This could involve starting with a 12-hour fasting window and gradually extending it as the body acclimates to the changes.

3. Nutrient-dense Eating: During eating windows, emphasis should be placed on consuming nutrient-dense, hormone-balancing foods such as leafy greens, lean proteins, healthy fats, and fiber-rich carbohydrates. These choices can help support hormonal balance and mitigate PMS symptoms.

4. Hydration and Electrolyte Balance: Adequate hydration and electrolyte balance are essential, especially during fasting periods. Maintaining these balances can help mitigate potential discomfort associated with fasting, ensuring a smoother transition into this dietary practice.

5. Mindful Eating: Incorporating mindfulness practices around food consumption can help women develop a healthier relationship with food and their bodies, potentially influencing their experience of PMS symptoms.

Embracing Intermittent Fasting as an Empowering Path to PMS Relief

In conclusion, the potential for intermittent fasting to alleviate PMS discomfort is an area ripe for exploration and application, particularly for women over 50 seeking to reclaim agency over their hormonal health. While further research is needed to delineate the precise mechanisms by which intermittent fasting exerts its effects on PMS symptoms, the existing body of evidence, coupled with the anecdotal experiences of many women, suggests promising avenues for relief.

By harnessing the science-backed strategies of intermittent fasting, women over 50 can take proactive steps towards mitigating the impact of PMS discomfort on their daily lives. Through a holistic approach encompassing tailored dietary choices, mindfulness practices, and informed lifestyle adjustments, intermittent fasting can serve as a valuable ally in the pursuit of hormonal balance and well-being. This empowering path holds the promise of not only alleviating PMS discomfort but also fostering a renewed sense of agency and vitality as women navigate the intricacies of perimenopause and beyond.

In the upcoming chapters, we will delve further into actionable meal plans, easy recipes, and lifestyle considerations, all designed to support women over 50 as they embrace the transformative potential of intermittent fasting in their journey towards hormonal balance and overall well-being.

Real-life Success Stories

The concept of **Intermittent Fasting for Hormonal Balance in Women Over 50** is multifaceted and compelling, especially when considering the tangible impact, it can have on women's lives. This sub-chapter, "Real-life Success Stories," represents the lived experiences of women who have embraced and found success through intermittent fasting Through their journeys, we gain insights, inspiration, and affirmation of the principles conveyed within this book.

In our quest to appreciate the power of intermittent fasting in the context of women over 50, we must lend our ears to the women who have traversed this path, faced various challenges, and emerged victorious in their pursuit of hormonal balance, PMS relief, perimenopause harmony, and weight management. Let these stories of real women spark a sense of hope, resilience, and determination within each reader, for the journey toward hormonal balance is indeed an individual odyssey, unique to each woman.

Real-life Success Stories: Women Over 50 Embracing Intermittent Fasting

Lila's Journey: Overcoming PMS and Finding Inner Harmony

Lila, a vibrant woman in her mid-50s, had always been an active proponent of natural health practices. However, when perimenopause engulfed her life with mood swings, fluctuating energy levels, and debilitating PMS symptoms, she felt lost. Traditional remedies and medications provided minimal relief, which eventually led Lila to explore new ways to manage her symptoms.

Upon discovering intermittent fasting as a potential solution to her hormonal imbalances, Lila decided to give it a try. With guidance from health professionals and the support of her community, she transitioned into a 16:8 fasting protocol. Gradually, she noticed subtle yet profound changes in her well-being. Her PMS symptoms lessened, her energy stabilized, and an overall sense of inner equilibrium started to unfold.

Lila's success story resonates with many women in their 50s who seek relief from the tumult of perimenopause. Her testimonial serves as a beacon of hope, reminding women that through mindful lifestyle adjustments such as intermittent fasting, a path toward hormonal harmony is indeed within reach.

Maria's Achievements: Empowering Weight Management Through Fasting

Maria, a resilient and determined woman in her late 50s, struggled with weight management during her perimenopausal journey. Despite her dedication to exercise and dietary adjustments, shedding excess pounds seemed like an insurmountable task. Frustrated, she delved into research about hormonally supportive strategies and stumbled upon intermittent fasting as a potential avenue.

Driven by her aspiration for a healthier lifestyle, Maria decided to integrate intermittent fasting into her routine. With the guidance of health professionals, she adopted a 20:4 fasting regimen and consciously tailored her meal plans to accommodate this new approach. Over time, the subtle shifts turned into substantial transformations: her weight stabilized, energy surged, and her outlook on her journey transformed.

Maria's commitment and success typify the untold narrative of many women over 50. Her triumph accentuates the potential of intermittent fasting as a scientifically supported tool for weight management and hormonal harmony during the perimenopausal phase.

Sofia's Transformation: A Journey to Hormonal Harmony

Sofia, a spirited woman approaching her 60s, grappled with the complex web of perimenopausal symptoms, including erratic moods, night sweats, and hormonal fluctuations that disrupted her overall well-being. Determined to seek a holistic approach, Sofia explored various options and eventually embraced intermittent fasting as part of her wellness plan.

By adhering to a 14:10 fasting pattern and enriching her dietary choices with hormone-balancing foods, Sofia nurtured a transformative journey. Her nights became more restful, her mental acuity improved, and her overall emotional state found newfound stability.

Sofia's story echoes the shared experiences of women approaching and navigating the perimenopausal tapestry. Her narrative exemplifies the potential for intermittent fasting to act as a catalyst for hormonal equilibrium, empowering women to reclaim control and harmony.

These real-life success stories underscore the transformative potential of intermittent fasting within the lives of women over 50. Through mindful adaptation and the sheer will to embrace change, these women have discovered renewed hope and balance amid the complexities of hormonal fluctuations. Their experiences are not just anecdotes; they are living testaments to the efficacy of intermittent fasting as a tool for hormonal balance and overall well-being.

As we resonate with these remarkable stories, let us harness the collective strength they exude. Let us draw inspiration from the victories of Lila, Maria, and Sofia and recognize that our journeys toward hormonal balance and well-being are not solitary endeavors. May these narratives infuse each reader with the resilience and determination needed to forge their distinct paths toward hormonal harmony, PMS relief, perimenopause tranquility, and weight management success through the science-backed strategies of intermittent fasting.

In embracing the power of intermittent fasting, as witnessed through these authentic narratives, may each reader kindle the flame of hope and possibility as they chart onward on their unique odyssey of transformation and hormonal equilibrium.

Chapter 5: Perimenopause Harmony and Intermittent Fasting

As women transition through the phases of life, the hormonal journey can be both challenging and transformative. For women over 50, perimenopause can usher in a range of physical and emotional changes, from fluctuating hormone levels to shifts in metabolism and weight management. In this pivotal chapter, we delve into the powerful intersection of perimenopause and intermittent fasting, uncovering the science-backed strategies that enable women to achieve hormonal balance, manage perimenopausal symptoms, and set out on a journey to achieve overall wellness.

Understanding Perimenopause: A Transformative Phase in a Woman's Life

Perimenopause, often referred to as the transitional phase leading to menopause, typically begins in a woman's 40s or 50s. During this time, the ovaries gradually produce less estrogen, leading to irregular menstrual cycles, fluctuations in hormone levels, and a myriad of symptoms that can significantly impact daily life. From hot flashes, night sweats, and mood swings to changes in libido, sleep disturbances, and weight gain, perimenopause encompasses a spectrum of experiences unique to each woman.

Moreover, the metabolic changes that accompany perimenopause can make weight management a formidable challenge. The decline in estrogen levels can influence how the body regulates weight, often leading to an increase in visceral fat and a decrease in muscle mass. As a result, women may find themselves facing an uphill battle when striving to maintain a healthy weight and metabolic equilibrium.

The Science of Intermittent Fasting: A Beacon of Hope for Hormonal Harmony

Intermittent fasting, a dietary approach focused on alternating periods of eating and fasting, has gained substantial recognition for its potential to address a multitude of health concerns, including weight management, metabolic health, and hormonal balance. The scientific foundation of intermittent fasting lies in the metabolic and cellular adaptations that occur during fasting periods, offering a promising avenue for women seeking to harmonize their hormone levels and navigate the challenges of perimenopause.

Research has illuminated the profound impact of intermittent fasting on various hormonal systems within the body. By modulating insulin sensitivity, reducing inflammation, and promoting cellular repair processes, intermittent fasting holds the potential to mitigate the symptoms of perimenopause while fostering overall well-being. Furthermore, intermittent fasting may support the maintenance of lean muscle mass and aid in the management of metabolic parameters, offering a comprehensive approach to address the multifaceted aspects of perimenopausal health.

Realizing Perimenopause Harmony Through Intermittent Fasting: Stories of Triumph and Transformation

Embedded within the tapestry of perimenopause are real-life success stories of women who have harnessed the potential of intermittent fasting to traverse this transformative phase with resilience and grace. Let's illuminate the narratives of these remarkable women, shedding light on the ways in which intermittent fasting has empowered them to realize hormonal harmony and reclaim control over their well-being.

Meet Susan: Navigating Hormonal Turbulence with Intermittent Fasting

Susan, a vibrant woman in her late 50s, found herself grappling with the myriad challenges of perimenopause. From erratic mood swings and disrupted sleep patterns to weight fluctuations and persistent fatigue, Susan's journey through perimenopause was marked by a sense of unyielding turbulence. Frustrated by the relentless impact of hormonal imbalances on her quality of life, Susan embarked on a quest to regain equilibrium and vitality.

Discovering intermittent fasting as a potential ally in her journey, Susan cautiously embraced this dietary strategy, seeking to recalibrate her hormonal landscape and revitalize her overall health. Emboldened by the research-backed promise of intermittent fasting in modulating hormonal balance, Susan initiated a structured approach, incorporating fasting periods and mindful meal planning into her daily routine.

Over time, Susan experienced a remarkable transformation. The practice of intermittent fasting, combined with a focus on nutrient-dense meals, not only supported Susan in managing her weight but also contributed to a tangible alleviation of perimenopausal symptoms. Her energy levels surged, mood stability improved, and she found herself navigating perimenopause with a newfound sense of resilience and composure.

Susan's journey stands as a testament to the potential of intermittent fasting in fostering hormonal harmony, empowering women to embrace perimenopause as a phase of growth and renewal.

Embracing Empowerment: The Path to Perimenopause Harmony and Beyond

The narratives of women like Susan showcase the profound impact of intermittent fasting as a catalyst for positive change amidst the realm of perimenopause. Their experiences embody the essence of empowerment, highlighting the transformative potential of embracing intentional lifestyle modifications and harnessing the innate resilience of the female body.

As we traverse the landscape of perimenopause and intermittent fasting, it becomes evident that the journey towards hormonal balance is far from solitary. It is intertwined with a nuanced tapestry of support systems, education, and a deep-rooted commitment to holistic well-being. By amalgamating the scientific underpinnings of intermittent fasting with the narratives of real-life success stories, women over 50 are encouraged to embark on a journey of self-discovery, resilience, and wellness.

The harmonious integration of intermittent fasting into the tapestry of perimenopause underscores the potential for transformative change, empowering women to reclaim agency over their health and well-being. As we navigate the intricate terrain of perimenopause and embrace the science-backed strategies of intermittent fasting, we pave the way for a future defined by resilience, vitality, and unwavering harmony, a future that embodies the essence of thriving amidst the beauty of transformation.

Navigating the Perimenopausal Phase with Hormonal Balance

As women enter the phase of perimenopause, which typically begins in their 40s or early 50s, they often experience a myriad of hormonal changes that can impact their physical, emotional, and mental well-being. These changes can bring about symptoms such as irregular periods, hot flashes, night sweats, mood swings, and disruptions in sleep patterns. It's crucial for women in this phase of life to understand and effectively navigate these changes to maintain their overall health and well-being.

This sub-chapter delves into the vital topic of "Navigating the Perimenopausal Phase with Hormonal Balance," which focuses on how intermittent fasting can be a science-backed strategy for supporting women in managing the symptoms of perimenopause. We will comprehensively explore the ways in which intermittent fasting can positively impact hormonal balance, provide relief from common perimenopausal symptoms, and support weight management in a manner specific to the needs of women over 50.

Understanding the Perimenopausal Phase

Before delving into the role of intermittent fasting, it's essential to understand the perimenopausal phase itself. Perimenopause is the transitional period leading to menopause, during which a woman's body gradually makes the natural transition to the end of her reproductive years. This phase is marked by fluctuating hormone levels, particularly estrogen and progesterone, leading to a range of physical and emotional changes.

One key aspect of perimenopause is the hormonal imbalance that can occur, ultimately impacting a woman's quality of life. As the body adapts to decreasing levels of estrogen, women may experience symptoms such as hot flashes, night sweats, mood swings, and irregular menstrual cycles. Furthermore, weight management can become more challenging due to hormonal shifts, potentially leading to increased visceral fat and changes in metabolism.

Recognizing the Impact of Hormonal Balance

Hormonal balance plays a pivotal role in the overall well-being of women, particularly during perimenopause. When hormones such as estrogen, progesterone, and testosterone are in harmony, women are more likely to experience regular menstrual cycles, better mood stability, and improved energy levels. Conversely, hormonal imbalances can lead to disruptive symptoms, including weight gain, mood disturbances, and sleep disturbances, impacting overall quality of life.

In addressing these changes, it's crucial to adopt strategies that support hormonal balance and mitigate the impact of these symptoms. This is where the concept of intermittent fasting comes into play as a science-backed approach that shows promise in promoting hormonal equilibrium, managing perimenopausal symptoms, and supporting healthy weight management.

Intermittent Fasting: A Science-Backed Strategy for Hormonal Balance

Intermittent fasting, characterized by alternating cycles of eating and fasting, has gained attention for its potential to positively influence hormonal balance and metabolic health. Research indicates that intermittent fasting may affect the body's hormone levels, including insulin, cortisol, and growth hormone, in ways that can be advantageous, particularly for women navigating through the perimenopausal phase.

Insulin Sensitivity and Blood Sugar Regulation

During perimenopause, women may experience fluctuations in insulin sensitivity and blood sugar regulation, which can contribute to weight gain and exacerbate symptoms such as hot flashes and mood swings. Intermittent fasting has been shown to enhance insulin sensitivity, potentially leading to better blood sugar control and decreased insulin resistance. By regulating insulin levels through intermittent fasting, women may experience improved overall well-being and better management of metabolic changes associated with perimenopause.

Impact on Growth Hormone and Metabolism

As women age, the decline in growth hormone production can lead to changes in metabolic rate and body composition. Intermittent fasting has been linked to an increase in growth hormone secretion, potentially contributing to enhanced fat metabolism and muscle preservation. This aspect of intermittent fasting is particularly relevant for women over 50 who are focused on managing weight and maintaining lean muscle mass during perimenopause.

Cortisol Regulation and Stress Management

The perimenopausal phase can also be characterized by increased stress levels and a heightened impact of cortisol, a hormone released in response to stress. Elevated cortisol levels can contribute to weight gain, particularly around the abdominal area, increased inflammation, and disrupted sleep patterns. Intermittent fasting, when practiced alongside stress-reducing techniques, may help in regulating cortisol levels and mitigating the adverse effects of stress, thereby supporting a more balanced hormonal environment.

Supportive Real-life Success Stories

To truly understand the impact of intermittent fasting on perimenopausal hormonal balance and overall well-being, real-life success stories are invaluable. Let's explore the experiences of women who have embraced intermittent fasting during their perimenopausal phase and have achieved meaningful results.

Lila's Journey to Hormonal Harmony

Lila, a 52-year-old woman, found herself struggling with debilitating hot flashes, low energy levels, and undesired weight gain as she entered perimenopause. Frustrated with the impact these symptoms were having on her daily life, she turned to intermittent fasting as a potential solution. With guidance from her healthcare provider, Lila adopted a 16:8 intermittent fasting approach, where she fasted for 16 hours and consumed her meals within an 8-hour window.

After consistently practicing intermittent fasting for several weeks, Lila began to notice substantial improvements. Her hot flashes became less frequent, and she experienced renewed energy levels during the day. Additionally, she found that her weight stabilized, and she felt more empowered to manage her overall well-being. Lila's success story serves as a testament to the potential of intermittent fasting in supporting hormonal balance and alleviating perimenopausal symptoms.

Amelia's Journey to Emotional Well-being

Amelia, a 48-year-old woman, grappled with mood swings, anxiety, and disrupted sleep patterns as she navigated through perimenopause. These emotional disturbances took a toll on her quality of life, causing her to seek out holistic approaches to address her symptoms. Upon discovering the potential benefits of intermittent fasting, Amelia decided to embark on a journey to integrate fasting into her lifestyle.

By gradually incorporating intermittent fasting, Amelia observed a remarkable shift in her emotional well-being. She reported feeling more emotionally stable, with reduced anxiety levels and improved sleep quality. This positive transformation in her mood and overall mental wellness significantly enhanced her ability to navigate through the perimenopausal phase with greater resilience and optimism.

These real-life success stories underscore the transformative potential of intermittent fasting in promoting hormonal balance, relieving perimenopausal symptoms, and supporting overall well-being for women over 50.

Science-backed Strategies for Implementing Intermittent Fasting

In light of the compelling real-life success stories and the scientific support for intermittent fasting as a strategy for perimenopausal harmony, it's crucial to explore practical and actionable approaches for integrating intermittent fasting into one's lifestyle. Consider the following science-backed strategies tailored to the unique needs of women over 50 as they navigate the perimenopausal phase:

Gradual Integration and Professional Guidance

When initiating intermittent fasting, it's important to start gradually and seek guidance from a healthcare provider, particularly for women with pre-existing health conditions. A gradual approach allows the body to acclimate to the fasting schedule, reducing the likelihood of potential discomfort or adverse effects. Consulting with a healthcare professional ensures that intermittent fasting aligns with individual health needs and provides tailored support throughout the process.

Adaptation to Circadian Rhythms

Women going through the perimenopausal phase may benefit from aligning their intermittent fasting schedule with their natural circadian rhythms. By incorporating an eating window that is in sync with their body's internal clock, women can optimize metabolic processes and hormonal function. This approach may enhance the overall effectiveness of intermittent fasting in promoting hormonal balance and metabolic health during perimenopause.

Nutrient-dense Meal Planning

During the eating window of intermittent fasting, it's essential for women over 50 to prioritize nutrient-dense, hormone-balancing meals that support hormonal health. Emphasizing a variety of whole foods, including lean proteins, healthy fats, and a colorful array of fruits and vegetables, can provide essential nutrients that bolster hormonal balance and overall well-being.

Incorporating Stress-reducing Practices

Given the potential impact of stress on hormonal balance, women in perimenopause can benefit from integrating stress-reducing practices alongside intermittent fasting. Techniques such as mindfulness, yoga, and deep breathing exercises can complement intermittent fasting by promoting cortisol regulation and fostering emotional resilience during this phase of life.

Empowering Through Knowledge and Support

Empowering women over 50 with accurate, evidence-based information about intermittent fasting and its potential benefits is a fundamental aspect of supporting their journey toward perimenopausal hormonal harmony. Providing a supportive environment and access to resources such as meal plans, recipes, and guidance from healthcare professionals can further enhance women's ability to embrace intermittent fasting as a sustainable and empowering strategy.

Empowering Women to Thrive in Perimenopause

The perimenopausal phase is a transformative period in a woman's life, marked by significant changes in hormonal balance and overall well-being. By harnessing the science-backed strategy of intermittent fasting, women over 50 can navigate through perimenopause with greater resilience, hormonal harmony, and empowered well-being. Real-life success stories, supported by scientific insights, illustrate the potential of intermittent fasting to alleviate perimenopausal symptoms, support hormonal balance, and foster overall health and vitality.

As we celebrate the triumphs of women who have embraced intermittent fasting and experienced meaningful changes in their well-being, it's crucial to acknowledge the empowerment that comes from understanding and navigating perimenopause with hormonal balance. By providing women with actionable strategies, comprehensive knowledge, and unwavering support, we empower them to thrive in perimenopause and embrace the transformative journey with vitality and resilience.

Intermittent Fasting Strategies for Perimenopausal Women

As women approach their 50s and beyond, perimenopause can bring about a host of hormonal changes that may impact their overall well-being. The transition into perimenopause is often accompanied by symptoms such as irregular periods, hot flashes, mood swings, and weight fluctuations. Intermittent fasting can serve as a powerful tool to support hormonal balance, manage weight, and alleviate some of the discomfort associated with perimenopause.

Understanding Perimenopause and Hormonal Fluctuations

Before diving into the specifics of intermittent fasting strategies for perimenopausal women, it's crucial to comprehend the hormonal shifts that occur during this phase of life. Perimenopause typically begins in a woman's 40s, although the exact timing varies from person to person. During perimenopause, the ovaries gradually produce less estrogen, leading to irregular menstrual cycles and other physical and emotional changes. Additionally, fluctuations in progesterone and testosterone levels can contribute to symptoms such as insomnia, fatigue, and mood disturbances.

The Impact of Intermittent Fasting on Hormonal Balance

Research has suggested that intermittent fasting can positively influence hormonal balance, particularly in women over 50. By engaging in strategic periods of fasting and eating, women can potentially mitigate some of the hormonal disruptions associated with perimenopause. Several key mechanisms underlie the beneficial effects of intermittent fasting on hormonal balance:

1. Insulin Sensitivity: Intermittent fasting has been shown to enhance insulin sensitivity, which is particularly beneficial for women experiencing age-related insulin resistance. Improving insulin sensitivity can help stabilize blood sugar levels and reduce the risk of developing conditions such as type 2 diabetes.

2. Growth Hormone Production: Fasting periods have been linked to an increase in growth hormone production, which plays a role in metabolism, muscle growth, and overall cellular repair. This can be especially beneficial for women navigating the metabolic changes that accompany perimenopause.

3. Cellular Repair and Autophagy: Intermittent fasting prompts a process known as autophagy, wherein cells remove damaged components and undergo repair processes. This cellular rejuvenation can support overall wellness and may be particularly advantageous for women experiencing age-related changes in cellular function.

4. Hormone Regulation: Some studies have suggested that intermittent fasting can influence the regulation of hormones such as leptin and ghrelin, which play a role in appetite control and metabolism. This regulation may

contribute to more stable energy levels and improved weight management during perimenopause.

Strategies for Implementing Intermittent Fasting in Perimenopause

While the benefits of intermittent fasting for perimenopausal women are compelling, it's essential to approach fasting strategies with mindfulness and consideration for individual needs. Here are science-backed intermittent fasting strategies tailored specifically for women over 50 navigating perimenopause:

1. Time-Restricted Eating: One of the most accessible approaches to intermittent fasting involves time-restricted eating, wherein individuals limit their daily eating window. For perimenopausal women, a common and manageable fasting window may involve fasting for 14-16 hours overnight, followed by an 8-10 hour eating window during the day. This approach aligns with the natural decline in metabolic rate that often occurs with age and can support weight management goals.

2. Alternate-Day Fasting: Another effective intermittent fasting strategy for perimenopausal women is alternate-day fasting. This approach involves alternating between days of regular eating and days of consuming significantly fewer calories, typically around 500-600 calories. When implemented thoughtfully, alternate-day fasting can contribute to weight management efforts and may offer metabolic benefits.

3. Modified Fasting Practices: Given the unique hormonal landscape of perimenopause, some women may benefit from modified fasting practices, such as the 5:2 method,

which involves eating normally for five days of the week and consuming fewer calories on two non-consecutive days. This approach allows for greater flexibility while still harnessing the potential benefits of intermittent fasting.

Addressing Potential Concerns and Considerations

It's important to approach intermittent fasting with an awareness of potential concerns and considerations specific to perimenopausal women. While the benefits of intermittent fasting are supported by scientific evidence, women over 50 should consider the following aspects when embarking on an intermittent fasting regimen:

1. Hormonal Health: Given the hormonal shifts occurring during perimenopause, it's crucial for women to monitor their individual responses to intermittent fasting and consult with healthcare providers as needed. Some women may find that certain fasting strategies impact their hormonal balance differently, emphasizing the importance of personalized approaches.

2. Nutrient Intake: As women age, nutrient needs may shift, and it's essential to ensure that intermittent fasting practices support adequate intake of essential nutrients. Incorporating nutrient-dense foods during eating windows and considering the use of dietary supplements can help address potential nutrient imbalances.

3. Stress Management: Perimenopause is a time of significant physical and emotional changes, and intermittent fasting should not contribute to excessive stress. Women should prioritize stress-reducing activities such as mindfulness practices, yoga, and adequate sleep to support overall well-being in conjunction with fasting practices.

4. Individualized Approach: Every woman's experience of perimenopause is unique, and thus, intermittent fasting strategies should be tailored to individual needs and preferences. Embracing flexibility and self-compassion while navigating intermittent fasting can contribute to a positive and sustainable experience.

Delicious Meal Plans and Recipes for Hormone-Balancing Success

Incorporating nutrient-rich, hormone-supportive meals into eating windows is pivotal for harnessing the full potential of intermittent fasting for perimenopausal women. The following meal plans and easy recipes are designed to complement intermittent fasting strategies and promote hormonal balance:

Meal Plan 1: Hormone-Supportive Breakfast Options

➢ Greek yogurt parfait with berries, chia seeds, and a drizzle of honey

➢ Whole-grain bread is paired with a spinach and feta omelet.

➢ Overnight oats with almond butter, sliced bananas, and a sprinkle of cinnamon

Meal Plan 2: Nourishing Lunch Ideas

➢ Quinoa salad with grilled chicken, mixed greens, cherry tomatoes, and a lemon-tahini dressing

➢ Lentil soup with a side of mixed greens and a whole-grain roll

➢ Grilled vegetable wrap with hummus, avocado, and a side of fresh fruit

Meal Plan 3: Satisfying Dinner Choices

➢ Baked salmon with roasted sweet potatoes and steamed broccoli

➢ Stir-fried vegetables and turkey over brown rice

➢ Spaghetti squash with marinara sauce, lean ground turkey, and a side of garlic spinach

Easy Recipes for Hormone-Balancing Snacks

➢ Roasted chickpeas tossed in olive oil and seasoned with paprika and cumin

➢ Nut butter drizzled over apple slices and sprinkled with hemp seeds

➢ Greek yogurt with a dollop of almond butter and a handful of mixed berries

By integrating these hormone-balancing meal plans and recipes into their eating patterns, perimenopausal women can support their overall health and well-being while practicing intermittent fasting.

Navigating perimenopause can present challenges and opportunities for women over 50, and leveraging the science-backed strategies of intermittent fasting can be a powerful tool in promoting hormonal balance, managing weight, and supporting overall wellness. By embracing time-restricted eating, alternate-day fasting, and modified fasting practices, women can adapt their intermittent fasting approach to align with the unique needs of perimenopause. Paired with thoughtful attention to hormonal health, nutrient intake, stress management, and individualized experiences, intermittent fasting can serve as a cornerstone in the journey toward hormonal harmony and well-being for perimenopausal women.

Lifestyle Changes to Support Hormonal Harmony

As women reach the age of 50 and beyond, their bodies undergo significant hormonal shifts, particularly during perimenopause. These changes can impact overall well-being, from mood swings and sleep disruptions to weight management challenges. Intermittent fasting is a powerful tool for addressing hormonal imbalances during this stage of life, but it works best when combined with supportive lifestyle changes. In this chapter, we will explore a range of lifestyle adjustments that can complement intermittent fasting for achieving hormonal harmony.

Understanding the Hormonal Landscape

Before delving into specific lifestyle changes, it's crucial to understand the hormonal landscape of perimenopause. Estrogen levels fluctuate, progesterone production declines, and the balance of other hormones such as testosterone and cortisol may also be affected. These hormonal changes can lead to symptoms like hot flashes, night sweats, fatigue, and mood swings, affecting the overall quality of life.

The Impact of Lifestyle on Hormonal Harmony

Embracing supportive lifestyle changes is pivotal in navigating the perimenopausal journey. Lifestyle modifications play a crucial role in managing symptoms and promoting overall well-being. By understanding the impact of these changes, women can empower themselves to navigate this phase of life with greater ease and vitality.

Dietary Strategies for Hormonal Balance

A well-balanced diet is a cornerstone of hormonal health. Including a variety of nutrient-dense foods can support hormone production, metabolism, and overall well-being. Integrating whole foods such as fruits, vegetables, lean proteins, and healthy fats into the diet can provide essential nutrients for hormonal harmony. Additionally, specific foods like flaxseeds, oily fish, and leafy greens can offer phytonutrients and omega-3 fatty acids that support hormone balance.

Physical Activity and Hormonal Balance

Regular physical activity offers myriad benefits for women experiencing perimenopause. Exercise can help manage weight, improve mood, and promote hormonal balance. Both aerobic activities and strength training can be particularly beneficial during this stage of life. Engaging in activities like yoga and Pilates can also aid in stress reduction and support overall hormonal harmony.

Managing Stress for Hormonal Well-being

The effects of stress on hormone balance should not be overlooked. Chronic stress can disrupt the intricate interplay of hormones, exacerbating symptoms of perimenopause. Implementing stress-reduction techniques such as meditation, deep breathing exercises, and mindfulness practices can be pivotal in promoting hormonal well-being. Adequate sleep is equally important, as it supports hormone regulation and overall vitality.

The Significance of Rest and Recover

Amidst the busyness of life, ensuring sufficient rest and recovery is essential for hormonal harmony. Prioritizing quality sleep and allowing for downtime can significantly impact hormone regulation. Establishing a consistent sleep schedule, creating a relaxing bedtime routine, and optimizing sleep environment are key strategies to support hormonal balance.

The Influence of Environmental Factors

Environmental factors can also impact hormonal health. Limiting exposure to endocrine-disrupting chemicals found in certain plastics, household products, and pesticides can promote hormonal harmony. Choosing organic products, using non-toxic cleaning supplies, and being mindful of personal care products can help minimize exposure to these potential disruptors.

Supportive Supplements for Hormonal Health

Supplements can complement a hormone-balancing lifestyle. Certain nutrients, such as vitamin D, magnesium, and B-complex vitamins, play essential roles in hormone synthesis and overall wellness. Incorporating these supplements, along with consultation with a healthcare provider, can support hormonal harmony.

In summary, cultivating lifestyle changes that support hormonal harmony is a vital component of navigating perimenopause with grace and vitality. Implementing a well-rounded approach inclusive of nutrition, physical activity, stress management, rest, environmental awareness, and supplements can empower women over 50 to embrace this stage of life with resilience and well-being. By integrating these lifestyle changes with intermittent fasting, women can harness the power of holistic strategies to promote hormonal balance and overall wellness.

Throughout this chapter, we have explored the multifaceted nature of lifestyle changes that can support hormonal harmony, with a particular focus on addressing the needs and challenges of women over 50. By fostering an environment that prioritizes hormonal balance, women can navigate perimenopause with greater ease, vitality, and resilience, paving the way for a life of holistic well-being and hormonal harmony.

Chapter 6
Intermittent Fasting for Weight Management

As we delve into Chapter 6 of our journey toward holistic wellness for women over 50, we're about to explore one of the most ubiquitous and versatile tools in the realm of health and well-being: intermittent fasting for weight management. This chapter is dedicated to showcasing how intermittent fasting can be a game-changer, offering a nuanced approach tailored specifically for the unique needs and experiences of perimenopausal women.

Understanding the Perimenopausal Journey

Before we plunge into the realm of intermittent fasting, it's essential to understand the incredible changes occurring in your body during perimenopause. This transitional phase, occurring typically in women between the ages of 45 and 55, is characterized by fluctuating hormone levels, irregular menstrual cycles, and a myriad of physical and emotional shifts. One of the most common experiences is weight gain and changes in body composition due to hormonal imbalances and a slowing metabolism.

Nurturing your body during this time is not just about losing weight but about empowering your body to function optimally, so you feel vibrant and strong throughout this transformative phase. As such, intermittent fasting presents itself as an eloquent strategy, addressing weight management coupled with hormone balance.

The Science Behind Intermittent Fasting

Intermittent fasting isn't a fad diet; it's a powerful tool entrenched in scientific research. It doesn't dictate what to eat but rather focuses on when to eat. The idea is to sync your meals with your body's natural rhythm, not only for weight management but also for optimizing hormone function and overall wellness.

When you fast, especially for extended periods, your body's insulin levels drop, allowing fat cells to release stored sugar for energy. Moreover, the process of intermittent fasting induces the cellular repair process of autophagy. This cleansing of cells supports healthy aging and reduces the risk of chronic diseases. Furthermore, intermittent fasting has been shown to help balance hormones such as insulin, ghrelin, and leptin, which play a crucial role in metabolism and weight management.

Tailored Intermittent Fasting for Perimenopausal Women

Understanding the nuanced needs of perimenopausal women, the approach to intermittent fasting for weight management may differ significantly from generic recommendations. Given the potential impact on hormone regulation, individualized and mindful strategies can make a world of difference. We'll explore some science-backed strategies tailored to address weight management specifically for perimenopausal women.

1. Time-restricted Eating

Time-restricted eating, a form of intermittent fasting, involves consuming all of your daily calories within a specific window of time. For perimenopausal women, a compressed eating window, such as 10-12 hours, helps regulate insulin levels, improve metabolic flexibility, and support weight management. This technique empowers your body to tap into fat stores during the fasting period while ensuring nourishment within a defined timeframe.

2. Fasting-Mimicking Diet

A fasting-mimicking diet involves following a low-calorie, plant-based meal plan for a few days each month. This approach may have particular relevance for women in perimenopause as it assists in regulating hormone levels, promoting cellular rejuvenation, and aiding healthy weight management. It's essential to work with a healthcare provider to personalize this approach to suit your unique needs.

3. Periodic Extended Fasting

Periodic extended fasting involves abstaining from food for longer stretches, typically 24-48 hours. This form of intermittent fasting triggers a deeper state of autophagy, which is vital for cleansing cells and enhancing metabolic health. This strategy, when pursued with care and guidance, can significantly contribute to weight management and hormonal harmony for perimenopausal women.

Mindful Eating and Enhanced Nutrient Intake

Intermittent fasting isn't just about when you eat; it also emphasizes what you eat. As a perimenopausal woman, your body requires nourishment that supports hormonal balance and overall well-being. Emphasize nutrient-dense foods, including plenty of vegetables, healthy fats, and lean protein sources. Additionally, consider incorporating specific nutrients such as omega-3 fatty acids, vitamin D, and antioxidants, which play a crucial role in hormone regulation and metabolic function during perimenopause.

Holistic Approach to Wellness

While intermittent fasting presents a potent strategy for weight management, it's vital to pair it with other holistic practices to support optimal well-being during perimenopause. Regular physical activity, adequate sleep, stress management, and mindfulness techniques all play critical roles in hormone regulation, weight management, and overall vitality. By weaving these elements together, you create a tapestry of wellness that harmonizes your body and mind, and empowers you to thrive during this phase of life.

Seeking Professional Guidance

Before embarking on any significant lifestyle changes, especially regarding eating patterns and fasting, it's essential to consult a qualified healthcare provider. Given the unique hormonal landscape of perimenopause, personalized guidance can help you tailor intermittent fasting strategies to align with your individual needs, ensuring you embark on this journey safely and with informed support.

Embracing Empowerment and Resilience

As we conclude our exploration of Chapter 6, it's essential to embrace the transformative power of intermittent fasting for weight management as a perimenopausal woman. This strategy isn't just about shedding pounds; it's about reclaiming agency over your well-being, nurturing your body, and fostering resilience during this profound phase of life. By incorporating tailored intermittent fasting strategies, aligning with mindful eating, and embracing a holistic approach to wellness, you pave the way toward hormonal harmony, weight management, and vibrancy that transcends your transition into menopause and beyond.

In our relentless pursuit of well-being, it's not just about the destination; it's about the journey the journey that pulsates with resilience, fortitude, and the unwavering spirit of women navigating the beautiful tapestry of life.

The Connection Between Hormones and Weight Gain After 50

As women age, many experiences hormonal changes that can impact their weight and overall well-being. After the age of 50, the body undergoes several hormonal shifts, particularly during perimenopause and menopause. These changes can often lead to weight gain and make it more challenging to maintain a healthy weight. Understanding the connection between hormones and weight gain after 50 is crucial in order to effectively manage these changes and maintain overall health.

Hormonal Changes After 50

When women reach their 50s, they often experience a significant decline in estrogen and progesterone levels as they approach menopause. Estrogen plays a key role in regulating metabolism and body weight. As its levels decrease, it can lead to changes in fat distribution and a decrease in lean body mass, which can contribute to weight gain and an increased risk of developing visceral adiposity, or "belly fat."

Furthermore, fluctuations in hormones such as insulin, cortisol, and thyroid hormones can occur, which can impact energy balance, appetite regulation, and the body's ability to manage stress. These hormonal changes can collectively contribute to weight gain and metabolic disturbances in women over 50.

The Impact of Hormonal Imbalance on Weight

Hormonal imbalance can lead to a variety of concerns related to weight gain after 50. For instance, insulin resistance might become more prevalent as women age, leading to increased fat storage, particularly in the abdominal area. This not only affects physical appearance but also increases the risk of developing chronic conditions such as type 2 diabetes and cardiovascular disease.

Additionally, the decline in estrogen levels can affect appetite and satiety regulation. Many women report an increase in cravings and feelings of hunger during perimenopause and menopause, which can lead to overeating and subsequent weight gain. The decrease in muscle mass and the natural slowdown of metabolism that accompanies aging can further compound these issues, making it more challenging to maintain a healthy weight.

Stress hormones such as cortisol can also play a role in weight management. Chronic stress, which is common among women managing family, career, and aging parents, can lead to increased production of cortisol, a hormone that, in excess, can contribute to weight gain, particularly around the midsection.

Scientific Insights into Hormonal Changes and Weight Management

Research has shown that hormone-related weight gain after 50 is a complex issue with multifaceted contributing factors. Understanding these underlying mechanisms can help women take proactive steps to manage their weight effectively. Intermittent fasting has emerged as a potential strategy to address the impact of hormonal changes on weight management during and after menopause.

Intermittent Fasting for Hormonal Balance and Weight Management

The eating pattern known as intermittent fasting (IF) alternates between times when one fasts and times when one eats. When done correctly, it can offer several benefits that specifically address the hormonal changes and weight management challenges faced by women over 50. Here's how intermittent fasting can positively impact hormonal balance and weight management:

1. Insulin Sensitivity: Intermittent fasting has been shown to improve insulin sensitivity, which is particularly important for women over 50 who may be at increased risk of developing insulin resistance. By enhancing insulin sensitivity, intermittent fasting can help the body better regulate blood sugar levels and reduce the risk of excess fat storage.

2. Hormonal Regulation: Intermittent fasting can influence hormonal balance, including insulin, ghrelin (the hunger hormone), and adiponectin, a hormone involved in regulating glucose levels and fatty acid breakdown. By optimizing these hormones, intermittent fasting can support healthier appetite regulation and fat metabolism, thereby contributing to weight management.

3. Metabolic Flexibility: Intermittent fasting promotes metabolic flexibility, allowing the body to efficiently switch between using glucose and fat for energy. This metabolic adaptation is particularly beneficial for women over 50 grappling with age-related metabolic changes. By

enhancing the body's ability to utilize stored fat for energy, intermittent fasting can support weight management.

4. Stress Reduction: Intermittent fasting has been linked to reduced levels of cortisol, the stress hormone. By managing cortisol levels, intermittent fasting can help mitigate the impact of chronic stress on weight gain, particularly around the midsection.

5. Cellular Repair and Longevity: Intermittent fasting triggers cellular repair processes such as autophagy, which help remove damaged cells and support overall cellular health. This can have a positive impact on aging-related hormonal changes and potentially support healthy weight management as women navigate their 50s and beyond.

Implementing Intermittent Fasting as a Lifestyle Approach

When considering intermittent fasting as a strategy for managing weight and hormonal balance after 50, it's important to approach it in a way that aligns with individual needs and preferences.

Starting with a moderate approach, such as the 16/8 method, can be a practical way to introduce intermittent fasting. This approach involves fasting for 16 hours, including the time spent sleeping, and then consuming all meals within an 8-hour window. It provides flexibility and can be adapted to suit different lifestyles.

The 5:2 method, which involves eating normally for five days a week and restricting calorie intake on the remaining two non-consecutive days, is another intermittent fasting approach that can be suitable for women over 50. This method may be particularly attractive to individuals who prefer a less restrictive fasting schedule.

The alternating day fasting approach, where individuals fast every other day or consume very few calories on fasting days, presents another option. While this method may yield rapid results, it's essential to consider individual tolerance and sustainability, especially for women navigating the complexities of hormonal changes and weight management after 50.

It's crucial to accompany intermittent fasting with a nutrient-dense, balanced diet that supports overall health and hormonal balance. Emphasizing whole foods, ample protein, healthy fats, and an abundance of fruits and vegetables can complement intermittent fasting to ensure optimal nutrient intake for women over 50.

Furthermore, incorporating regular physical activity and strength training into a lifestyle focused on intermittent fasting can help preserve lean muscle mass, promote bone health, and support metabolic function. These lifestyle elements are crucial for effective weight management and overall well-being.

Consulting with a healthcare provider or a registered dietitian can offer personalized guidance and support, particularly for women over 50 who may have specific health concerns or dietary considerations. Working with a knowledgeable professional can help tailor an intermittent fasting plan to individual needs and ensure it complements overall health and hormonal balance.

The Psychological and Emotional Aspect

Managing weight and navigating hormonal changes after 50 can also have a significant emotional and psychological impact. It's essential for women to approach these changes with self-compassion and to cultivate a positive relationship with food, body image, and aging.

Practicing mindfulness, engaging in stress-reducing activities, and seeking social support can all contribute to a holistic approach to managing hormonal changes and weight after 50. By addressing the emotional aspects of these transitions, women can foster a more supportive environment for sustainable and successful weight management.

The connection between hormones and weight gain after 50 is a multifaceted issue that requires a comprehensive approach. Intermittent fasting has emerged as a potential strategy to support hormonal balance and effective weight management for women navigating the complexities of perimenopause, menopause, and beyond. By understanding the impact of hormonal changes on weight and implementing evidence-based lifestyle strategies, women over 50 can empower themselves to manage their well-being proactively.

As with any significant lifestyle change, it's crucial for women to consult with healthcare professionals and trusted experts to develop a personalized approach that aligns with their individual needs, preferences, and health considerations. With the right support and knowledge, women can navigate the challenges of hormonal changes and weight management after 50 with resilience, grace, and a focus on overall health and well-being.

Intermittent Fasting as a Tool for Sustainable Weight Loss

Navigating the journey of weight management can be a complex and daunting task, especially for women over 50. This pivotal stage in life brings with it unique hormonal fluctuations that can make sustainable weight loss seem like an elusive goal. However, within the realm of scientifically validated strategies, intermittent fasting emerges as a powerful tool for not only promoting hormonal balance but also achieving sustainable weight loss. In this chapter, we will dive deep into the world of intermittent fasting and explore how it can be harnessed as a sustainable approach to shedding excess weight and promoting overall well-being in the context of hormone balance for women over 50.

Understanding Intermittent Fasting

Intermittent fasting, often abbreviated as IF, is not a diet in the traditional sense. Instead, it is an eating pattern that cycles between periods of eating and fasting. The focus is not on what to eat, but rather when to eat. There are several popular methods of intermittent fasting, each with its unique approach to the fasting and eating windows. Some of the most commonly practiced methods include the 16/8 method, the 5:2 diet, Eat-Stop-Eat, and the alternate-day fasting.

The 16/8 method involves restricting eating to an 8-hour window, followed by a 16-hour fasting period. The 5:2 diet suggests consuming a standard diet for five days of the week, and then limiting caloric intake to 500-600 calories on the remaining two non-consecutive days. Eat-Stop-Eat involves fasting for 24 hours once or twice a week, while the alternate-day fasting method alternates between normal eating days and fasting days.

While the mechanisms behind intermittent fasting are multifaceted, one of the primary reasons it is effective for sustainable weight loss is its impact on insulin levels. When we eat, especially foods high in carbohydrates, our body releases insulin to help regulate blood sugar levels. However, consistently high insulin levels can lead to insulin resistance, which is often associated with weight gain and metabolic disorders. Intermittent fasting helps lower insulin levels during fasting periods, thereby promoting fat burning and making stored body fat more accessible for energy.

Another key aspect of intermittent fasting is its potential to increase levels of norepinephrine, a hormone and neurotransmitter that plays a role in the body's fight-or-flight response. Increased norepinephrine levels can lead to higher metabolic rate and enhanced fat burning, further contributing to sustainable weight loss.

Impact of Intermittent Fasting on Hormonal Balance

In the context of women over 50, hormonal balance is of paramount importance not only for weight management but also for overall well-being. The fluctuations in estrogen, progesterone, and testosterone levels during perimenopause and menopause can pose significant challenges to maintaining a healthy weight. Additionally, imbalances in hormones such as insulin and cortisol can further complicate the weight loss journey.

This is where intermittent fasting emerges as a powerful ally in restoring hormonal balance. Research indicates that intermittent fasting can have a positive impact on several key hormones, including insulin, ghrelin, leptin, and cortisol. By modulating these hormones, intermittent fasting can help improve insulin sensitivity, reduce hunger cravings, and optimize fat-burning processes, ultimately supporting sustainable weight loss in women over 50.

In particular, intermittent fasting has been shown to decrease insulin resistance, which is a common issue during perimenopause and menopause. As insulin sensitivity improves, the body becomes more efficient at utilizing nutrients for energy, which can aid in weight management and reduce the risk of developing metabolic disorders such as type 2 diabetes.

Furthermore, intermittent fasting can influence ghrelin and leptin levels, two hormones that play crucial roles in regulating hunger and satiety. By reducing ghrelin, the hormone that stimulates hunger, and increasing leptin, the hormone that signals fullness, intermittent fasting can help women over 50 achieve better control over their appetite and food intake, leading to sustainable weight loss outcomes.

Practical Considerations and Implementation of Intermittent Fasting

While the science behind intermittent fasting is compelling, the practical implementation of this eating pattern requires a thoughtful approach, especially for women over 50. It is essential to underscore that intermittent fasting is not suitable for everyone, and individual factors such as existing medical conditions, medications, and nutritional needs should be taken into account before embarking on an intermittent fasting regimen.

For women over 50 considering intermittent fasting as a tool for sustainable weight loss, it is crucial to consult with a healthcare provider or a qualified nutrition professional to assess individual health status and determine the most appropriate fasting method. Additionally, incorporating nutrient-dense whole foods, lean proteins, healthy fats, and adequate hydration during eating windows is essential to support overall health and well-being.

Moreover, it is important to approach intermittent fasting with a mindset of self-care and self-awareness. Listening to one's body signals and making gradual adjustments to the fasting and eating windows can help in creating a sustainable and personalized intermittent fasting routine. Furthermore, combining intermittent fasting with regular physical activity tailored to individual needs and abilities can amplify the benefits of this approach to sustainable weight loss for women over 50.

Empowering women over 50 with the knowledge and tools needed to embrace intermittent fasting as a sustainable strategy for weight management is a transformative endeavor. By understanding the scientific principles underlying intermittent fasting and its potential impact on hormonal balance, women can cultivate a renewed sense of agency and empowerment in their journey towards sustainable weight loss and overall well-being.

Intermittent fasting stands as a testament to the remarkable intersection between science-backed strategies for sustainable weight loss and the promotion of hormonal balance in women over 50. By harnessing the power of intermittent fasting, women in this demographic can embark on a transformative path towards achieving their weight management goals while prioritizing their overall health and well-being.

As we conclude this exploration of intermittent fasting as a tool for sustainable weight loss, it is crucial to emphasize the importance of mindful and informed decision-making. Embracing intermittent fasting as a sustainable approach to weight loss requires a holistic understanding of its potential benefits and implications, along with a commitment to self-care and self-awareness. By approaching this journey with curiosity, resilience, and a spirit of empowerment, women over 50 can unlock the transformative potential of intermittent fasting in their pursuit of sustainable weight management and hormonal balance.

Balancing Nutrition for Optimal Results

As a woman over 50, achieving and maintaining optimal health and well-being is a top priority. In the quest for hormonal balance and sustainable weight management, nutrition plays a pivotal role. In this comprehensive guide, we'll delve into the art of balancing nutrition for optimal results, specifically tailored for the unique needs of women over 50 engaging in intermittent fasting to support hormonal harmony and weight management.

Understanding the Foundations of Nutrition

Nutrition is the cornerstone of overall health. For women navigating the challenges of perimenopause and beyond, it becomes increasingly critical to pay attention to the quality of the food consumed. Balancing nutrition involves ensuring that your body receives the necessary nutrients while avoiding excessive intake of less healthy substances.

Key Nutrients for Women Over 50

As women transition through menopause and beyond, the body's nutrient needs change. Calcium and vitamin D become even more crucial to support bone health and reduce the risk of osteoporosis. Omega-3 fatty acids can alleviate symptoms related to menopause, such as joint pain and inflammation, while also supporting heart health. Additionally, maintaining a diet rich in antioxidants, fiber, and protein is vital for overall well-being.

The Role of Macronutrients

Macronutrients—carbohydrates, proteins, and fats—are the primary components of our diet, and their proportions matter significantly. Carbohydrates, especially whole grains, fruits, and vegetables, provide essential energy and fiber. Proteins are the building blocks for body tissue, supporting muscle and bone health. Fats, especially healthy fats like those found in avocados, nuts, and oily fish, are essential for hormone production and overall cellular function.

Tailoring Nutrition to Support Intermittent Fasting

Intermittent fasting can be a powerful tool for women over 50 seeking hormonal balance and sustainable weight management. When combined with a balanced and nutritious diet, it holds the potential to revolutionize health outcomes. However, to maximize its benefits, it's paramount to pay attention to the nutritional composition of meals during both eating and fasting windows.

Break the Fast with Balanced Nutrition

The first meal after fasting, often referred to as "breaking the fast," can set the tone for the day. Optimal nutrition in this meal is pivotal. A balance of macronutrients is crucial, as it helps stabilize blood sugar levels and kick-starts the metabolism. Incorporating lean proteins, healthy fats, and complex carbohydrates can provide sustained energy while supporting muscle maintenance and overall satiety.

Prioritizing Nutrient-Dense Foods

Within the eating window, emphasizing nutrient-dense foods becomes paramount. This includes a variety of colorful fruits and vegetables, lean proteins, whole grains, and healthy fats. Nutrient-dense foods are rich in essential vitamins and minerals, providing the body with the necessary tools for optimal function and helping to promote overall well-being.

Hydration and Nutrient Absorption

Proper hydration is often overlooked but is a vital aspect of nutrient absorption, especially for women over 50. Staying well-hydrated supports digestion, circulation, and the transportation of nutrients throughout the body. For optimal results, ensuring adequate water intake and incorporating hydrating foods such as cucumbers, watermelon, and leafy greens can support overall health.

Optimizing Nutrient Absorption for Hormonal Harmony

Fluctuating hormone levels can impact how the body processes and absorbs nutrients. To support hormonal balance, tailoring nutrition strategies becomes even more critical. Understanding how specific nutrients interact with hormone regulation can empower women over 50 to optimize their dietary choices for hormonal harmony.

Phytonutrients and Hormonal Balance

Phytonutrients, found in colorful fruits and vegetables, have been shown to support hormonal balance. For instance, cruciferous vegetables like broccoli and kale contain compounds that aid in estrogen metabolism, potentially reducing the risk of estrogen dominance. Similarly, foods rich in flavonoids, such as berries and citrus fruits, can help regulate hormonal fluctuations.

Gut Health and Hormonal Balance

The gut microbiome plays a fundamental role in hormone regulation and overall well-being. Incorporating probiotic-rich foods like yogurt, kefir, and fermented vegetables can support gut health, potentially aiding in estrogen metabolism and promoting hormonal balance. Additionally, consuming prebiotic foods, such as garlic, onions, and bananas, can nourish beneficial gut bacteria, further supporting hormonal harmony.

Omega-3 Fatty Acids and Inflammation

Inflammation can exacerbate hormonal imbalances, contributing to symptoms such as bloating and joint pain. Omega-3 fatty acids, found in fatty fish, chia seeds, and flaxseeds, possess anti-inflammatory properties, potentially alleviating discomfort associated with hormonal fluctuations. By prioritizing omega-3-rich foods, women over 50 can actively support their bodies in managing inflammation and promoting overall well-being.

Antioxidants and Cellular Health

As women age, cellular health becomes increasingly crucial for overall vitality. Antioxidant-rich foods, including berries, dark chocolate, and green tea, can combat oxidative stress, potentially protecting cells from damage related to hormonal changes. By including a variety of antioxidant sources in their diet, women over 50 can actively support their cellular health and potentially mitigate the impact of hormonal fluctuations.

Practical Strategies for Balancing Nutrition

Meal Planning and Preparation

Planning and preparing meals in advance can streamline the process of maintaining balanced nutrition while practicing intermittent fasting. By incorporating a variety of nutrient-dense foods into meal plans, women over 50 can ensure they receive essential nutrients while supporting their overall health and wellness goals.

Mindful Eating and Nutrient Absorption

Practicing mindful eating techniques, such as chewing slowly and savoring each bite, can facilitate optimal nutrient absorption. By being present and attuned to their meals, women over 50 can enhance the digestive process, potentially improving nutrient uptake and overall satisfaction from meals.

Seeking Professional Guidance

For women over 50 navigating the complexities of nutrition, seeking guidance from a registered dietitian or nutritionist can provide personalized insights and support. A professional can tailor dietary recommendations to individual needs, helping women optimize their nutrition for hormonal balance and sustainable well-being.

Balancing nutrition for optimal results is a multifaceted endeavor, especially for women over 50 focusing on intermittent fasting to support hormonal harmony and weight management. By prioritizing nutrient-dense foods, supporting hydration, and tailoring dietary choices to promote hormonal balance, women can harness the power of nutrition to enhance their overall well-being. Embracing science-backed strategies for nutrient optimization empowers women over 50 to cultivate sustainable health and vitality as they navigate the transformative journey of hormonal balance and intermittent fasting.

Incorporating these insights into daily life can profoundly impact not only hormonal balance and weight management but also overall well-being, setting the stage for long-term health and vitality.

Chapter 7: Delicious Meal Plans for Hormonal-Balancing Success

In the quest for hormonal balance and overall health in women over 50, meal planning plays a pivotal role. This crucial aspect of intermittent fasting requires careful attention and consideration. In this chapter, we will delve into the intricacies of crafting delicious and nutritious meal plans to support hormonal balance, manage weight effectively, and ensure overall well-being for women in this significant phase of life.

Understanding the Needs of Women Over 50

As women reach the age of 50 and beyond, hormonal fluctuations become a prominent feature of their lives. The onset of perimenopause and menopause brings about significant changes in the body's hormonal landscape. These changes can lead to symptoms such as hot flashes, mood swings, weight gain, and disrupted sleep patterns. Understanding these challenges is essential in devising meal plans that alleviate these symptoms and promote hormonal balance.

Nutritional Requirements for Hormonal Balance

The nutritional needs of women over 50 are unique and require specific attention. Essential nutrients such as calcium, vitamin D, and magnesium become increasingly important to support bone health during this phase. Additionally, maintaining stable blood sugar levels and managing insulin sensitivity become pivotal for weight management and overall well-being.

Crafting Balanced and Nutrient-Dense Meal Plans

When creating meal plans for women over 50, it is crucial to focus on nutrient-density and balanced macronutrient composition. Incorporating a variety of colorful fruits and vegetables ensures an adequate intake of vitamins, minerals, and phytonutrients essential for hormonal balance. Lean `sources of protein, such as poultry, fish, and plant-based proteins, play a crucial role in supporting muscle mass and metabolic function.

Moreover, healthy fats derived from sources like avocados, nuts, and olive oil are valuable for hormonal health and cognitive function. These fats aid in the absorption of fat-soluble vitamins and contribute to satiety. Whole grains and complex carbohydrates provide sustained energy and fiber, supporting digestive health and stable blood sugar levels, thereby aiding in weight management.

Addressing Hormonal Imbalances Through Nutrition

Certain foods possess the unique ability to support hormone balance in women over 50. For instance, incorporating flaxseeds, which are rich in lignans, can aid in mitigating menopausal symptoms due to their potential estrogenic effects. Cruciferous vegetables such as broccoli, kale, and Brussels sprouts contain compounds that support estrogen metabolism, playing a role in hormonal harmony.

Additionally, including omega-3 fatty acids from sources like fatty fish and walnuts can help alleviate inflammation and promote cardiovascular health, which is especially crucial during menopausal years. These nutritional strategies can be integrated into delicious and satisfying meal plans, allowing women over 50 to navigate this phase of life with vitality and balance.

Supporting Hormonal Health Through Culinary Creativity

Delicious meal plans for hormonal balance should not only be nutritious but also enjoyable. Engaging the senses and exploring a variety of flavors and textures can make the transition to intermittent fasting and optimized nutrition an inspiring journey. By incorporating herbs and spices such as turmeric, ginger, and cinnamon, meal plans can offer anti-inflammatory and metabolism-boosting properties, enhancing overall health.

Furthermore, exploring global cuisines can introduce women to a diverse array of ingredients that offer unique health benefits. For example, incorporating fermented foods like kimchi and sauerkraut supports gut health, which is essential for overall immunity and hormonal balance. Additionally, embracing the richness of Mediterranean cuisine with its emphasis on olive oil, whole grains, and abundant fruits and vegetables offers a flavorful and healthful approach to meal planning.

Practical Tips for Meal Preparation and Planning

Meal planning can be simplified and made more efficient through strategic approaches. Utilizing batch cooking techniques allows for the preparation of nutritious components that can be combined in various ways throughout the week. Preparing versatile elements such as roasted vegetables, lean proteins, and whole grains enables the creation of diverse and balanced meals without repetitive cooking.

Furthermore, involving women in the meal planning process and encouraging them to take ownership of their nutritional choices can enhance their commitment to the journey of hormonal balance and well-being. This participatory approach allows for the customization of meal plans based on individual preferences and dietary requirements, fostering a sense of empowerment and control over one's health.

In the realm of intermittent fasting for hormonal balance in women over 50, the cultivation of delicious and well-rounded meal plans is a key determinant of success. From understanding the unique nutritional needs of this demographic to crafting flavorful and supportive meal options, the journey towards hormonal-balance and vitality is enriched through conscientious and creative meal planning. By embracing the art of culinary nourishment, women over 50 can discover the joy and empowerment of hormonally-balancing meal plans that nurture body, mind, and spirit.

Sample Meal Plans Tailored for Women Over 50

As women age, hormonal shifts can significantly impact their overall health and wellbeing. To address these changes and support hormonal balance, adopting a strategic approach to nutrition becomes increasingly important. Coupled with the practice of intermittent fasting, tailored meal plans can play a crucial role in supporting women over 50 on their journey towards optimal health and hormonal balance.

In the pursuit of health and wellness, women over 50 often seek effective strategies that not only support their physical health but also address the unique hormonal changes they experience. Understanding the impact of nutrition and intermittent fasting on hormonal balance is key to maintaining overall wellbeing and managing weight effectively. This chapter will delve into sample meal plans specifically tailored for women over 50, considering their nutritional needs, hormonal fluctuations, and overall health goals.

Balancing Nutritional Needs

Women's nutritional demands change significantly as they get older. The hormonal fluctuations associated with perimenopause and menopause often lead to a decrease in muscle mass, a slower metabolic rate, and changing nutrient requirements. Moreover, the risk of developing conditions such as osteoporosis, heart disease, and insulin resistance may increase. Hence, the importance of a well-balanced diet tailored to meet these changing needs cannot be overstated.

Sample Meal Plans

Incorporating intermittent fasting into the dietary regimen of women over 50 requires a thoughtful approach, ensuring that it aligns with their specific nutritional demands and health goals. Below are sample meal plans specially curated to support hormonal balance and overall health among women in this demographic:

Day 1: Hormone-Balancing Breakfast

- ➢ Spinach and feta omelet
- ➢ 1 slice of whole grain toast
- ➢ 1 cup of mixed berries

Intermittent Fasting Period

> ➤ Water, herbal tea, or black coffee

Day 1: Hormone-Balancing Lunch

> ➤ Grilled salmon fillet
> ➤ Quinoa and vegetable salad with a lemon vinaigrette dressing
> ➤ Steamed broccoli

Day 1: Hormone-Balancing Dinner

> ➤ Baked chicken breast
> ➤ Mixed green salad with olive oil and balsamic vinegar
> ➤ Roasted sweet potatoes

Day 2: Hormone-Balancing Breakfast

> ➤ Greek yogurt with chopped almonds and a sprinkle of honey
> ➤ 1 serving of chia seed pudding
> ➤ Herbal tea

Intermittent Fasting Period

> ➤ Water, herbal tea, or black coffee

Day 2: Hormone-Balancing Lunch

> ➤ Lentil and vegetable soup
> ➤ Whole grain roll
> ➤ Mixed fruit salad

Day 2: Hormone-Balancing Dinner

> ➤ Grilled shrimp skewers
> ➤ Quinoa pilaf
> ➤ Roasted asparagus

These sample meal plans prioritize nutrient-dense foods, lean proteins, healthy fats, and complex carbohydrates, catering to the specific dietary requirements of women over 50. Furthermore, the incorporation of intermittent fasting is intended to optimize hormonal balance, manage weight effectively, and support overall health.

Adapting Meal Plans to Individual Needs

It's important to recognize that individual nutritional requirements can vary widely. Factors such as activity levels, food preferences, and underlying health conditions should be taken into account when crafting personalized meal plans. Consulting with a qualified healthcare professional or registered dietitian can provide valuable insights and guidance tailored to specific needs and goals.

Sample meal plans tailored for women over 50, combined with the practice of intermittent fasting, can serve as a foundational component in achieving hormonal balance, managing weight, and supporting overall health. By emphasizing nutrient-rich foods, mindful eating, and strategic fasting periods, women in this demographic can attain a greater sense of wellness and vitality as they embrace the journey of aging gracefully and healthfully.

In summary, these sample meal plans are designed to be not only delicious and satisfying but also supportive of the unique nutritional needs of women over 50. With a focus on optimizing hormonal balance and overall health, these meal plans aim to empower women in this demographic to take charge of their well-being and embrace a holistic approach to health.

This comprehensive and science-backed approach to nutrition and intermittent fasting aims to equip women over

50 with practical strategies for maintaining optimal health, managing weight effectively, and nurturing hormonal balance.

By providing women in this demographic with tailored meal plans, we aim to support their journey toward hormonal balance, overall wellness, and sustained health as they embrace the age of 50 and beyond.

Nutrient-Dense Foods to Support Hormonal Health

Maintaining hormonal balance is crucial for women over 50, especially as they navigate the natural changes associated with perimenopause and menopause. Nutrition plays a vital role in supporting hormonal health during this stage of life. In this chapter, we will explore the importance of nutrient-dense foods and their impact on hormonal balance in women over 50. We will delve into the specific nutrients, food groups, and dietary strategies that can aid in supporting hormonal health and overall well-being.

The Significance of Nutrient-Dense Foods for Hormonal Health

As women age, hormonal fluctuations often become more pronounced. These changes can lead to symptoms such as hot flashes, mood swings, weight gain, and disrupted sleep patterns. Proper nutrition, particularly the consumption of nutrient-dense foods, can play a pivotal role in managing these symptoms and supporting hormonal balance.

Understanding Nutrient Density

Nutrient-dense foods are those that provide a high concentration of essential nutrients relative to their calorie content. These nutrients include vitamins, minerals, antioxidants, and phytochemicals that are vital for maintaining overall health and well-being. For women over 50, prioritizing nutrient-dense foods can help address specific nutritional needs while supporting hormonal balance.

Essential Nutrients for Hormonal Health

5. Calcium and Vitamin D: Adequate intake of calcium and vitamin D is essential for maintaining bone health and reducing the risk of osteoporosis, a common concern for women in postmenopausal years. Dairy products, leafy green vegetables, and fortified plant-based milk are excellent sources of calcium, while vitamin D is synthesized through exposure to sunlight. Additionally, vitamin D supports immune function and may have a role in hormone regulation.

6. Omega-3 Fatty Acids: Found in fatty fish, flaxseeds, chia seeds, and walnuts, omega-3 fatty acids offer anti-inflammatory properties and support cardiovascular health. They may also help alleviate symptoms of menopause, such as hot flashes and joint pain, while contributing to overall hormonal balance.

7. Phytoestrogens: Plant-based compounds with estrogenic activity, phytoestrogens can mimic the hormone estrogen in the body. Sources of phytoestrogens include soy products, flaxseeds, and legumes. These compounds may help alleviate menopausal symptoms by modulating estrogen levels in the body.

8. Magnesium: Magnesium plays a crucial role in numerous physiological processes, including muscle function, nerve function, and bone health. It also supports the body's

stress response and may help alleviate symptoms of anxiety and irritability often experienced during perimenopause and menopause. Whole grains, nuts, seeds, and dark leafy greens are good providers of magnesium.

9. Fiber: Adequate fiber intake from fruits, vegetables, whole grains, and legumes supports gut health and regular bowel movements. Fiber also assists in managing weight and may help control blood sugar levels, which is particularly important for women over 50 at risk of insulin resistance and type 2 diabetes.

Incorporating Nutrient-Dense Foods into Meal Plans

Crafting meal plans that prioritize nutrient-dense foods is a practical and effective approach for women over 50 looking to support hormonal health. Here, we present a sample meal plan tailored to the nutritional needs of women in this demographic:

Sample Meal Plan

Breakfast

- ➤ Berries and chia seeds sprinkled on top of Greek yogurt
- ➤ Whole grain toast with almond butter
- ➤ Herbal tea or water

Mid-Morning Snack

- ➤ Sliced apple with a handful of almonds

Lunch

> ➢ Grilled salmon salad with mixed greens, avocado, and a balsamic vinaigrette
> ➢ Quinoa or brown rice pilaf
> ➢ Herbal tea or water

Afternoon Snack

> ➢ Carrot sticks with hummus

Dinner

> ➢ Baked chicken breast with roasted vegetables (broccoli, cauliflower, carrots)
> ➢ Steamed asparagus
> ➢ Whole grain roll
> ➢ Herbal tea or water

Evening Snack

> ➢ Plain, unsweetened yogurt with a drizzle of honey

This carefully planned meal structure incorporates a variety of nutrient-dense foods, including lean protein sources, healthy fats, whole grains, and ample servings of fruits and vegetables. It also emphasizes hydration with herbal teas and water. Such a meal plan provides essential nutrients while promoting hormonal balance, bone health, and overall well-being.

Actionable Steps for Embracing Nutrient-Dense Eating

Beyond structured meal plans, there are several actionable steps women over 50 can take to embrace nutrient-dense eating and support hormonal health:

10. Mindful Eating: Paying attention to hunger cues and practicing mindful eating can help regulate portion sizes and prevent overeating. Mindful eating involves savoring each bite, chewing slowly, and appreciating the sensory experience of meals.

11. Diverse Vegetable Intake: Aim to consume a wide variety of vegetables, incorporating different colors and types to ensure a broad spectrum of vitamins, minerals, and phytonutrients.

12. Regular Physical Activity: Engaging in regular physical activity supports overall health and may assist in managing weight, alleviating stress, and promoting hormonal balance. Activities such as walking, yoga, and strength training can be particularly beneficial.

13. Hydration: Staying adequately hydrated is essential for hormonal health and overall well-being. Aim to drink plenty of water and incorporate herbal teas and infused water for variety.

14. Whole Foods Emphasis: Prioritize whole, minimally processed foods over highly refined and packaged products. Whole foods retain their natural nutrient content and are typically rich in essential vitamins and minerals.

Nutrient-dense foods play a pivotal role in supporting hormonal health and overall well-being for women over 50. By incorporating a range of essential nutrients, embracing diverse and balanced meals, and prioritizing whole foods, women can take proactive steps toward hormone balance, bone health, and managing the symptoms associated with perimenopause and menopause. Through informed dietary choices and mindful eating habits, women over 50 can empower themselves to navigate this stage of life with vitality and resilience.

Recipes for Hormone-Balancing Meals

For women over 50, maintaining hormonal balance through nutrition is crucial. Here are 20 different and unique recipes designed to support hormonal health, accompanied by nutritional information, ingredients, and preparation steps.

1. Quinoa and Vegetable Stir-Fry

Nutritional Information:

- Calories: 320 kcal
- Carbohydrates: 44g
- Protein: 12g
- Fat: 10g

Ingredients:

- 1 cup quinoa
- Two cups of mixed veggies, such as carrots, broccoli, and bell peppers
- 1 tbsp olive oil
- garlic cloves, minced

Preparation:

- As directed on the package, prepare the quinoa.
- In a pan, sauté vegetables with olive oil and garlic until tender.
- Toss vegetables with quinoa and season to taste.

2. Salmon and Asparagus Salad

Nutritional Information:

- Calories: 380 kcal
- Carbohydrates: 12g
- Protein: 28g
- Fat: 24g

Ingredients:

- 1 salmon fillet
- 2 cups asparagus, trimmed
- 2 tbsp balsamic vinaigrette
- Mixed greens

Preparation:

- Grill or bake seasoned salmon until cooked through.
- Steam asparagus until tender-crisp.
- Combine asparagus, salmon, and mixed greens. Drizzle with balsamic vinaigrette.

3. Mango and Turmeric Smoothie

Nutritional Information:

- Calories: 240 kcal
- Carbohydrates: 45g
- Protein: 8g
- Fat: 5g

Ingredients:

- 1 ripe mango, peeled and cubed
- 1 cup Greek yogurt
- 1 tsp turmeric
- ½ cup almond milk

Preparation:

> ➢ Blend all ingredients until smooth. Adjust consistency with almond milk as desired.

4. Eggplant and Chickpea Curry

Nutritional Information:

> ➢ Calories: 290 kcal
> ➢ Carbohydrates: 38g
> ➢ Protein: 10g
> ➢ Fat: 12g

Ingredients:

> ➢ 1 large eggplant, diced
> ➢ 1 can chickpeas, drained
> ➢ 1 cup coconut milk
> ➢ 2 tbsp curry powder

Preparation:

> ➢ Sauté eggplant and chickpeas in olive oil.
> ➢ Add curry powder and coconut milk. Simmer until eggplant is tender.

5. Sweet Potato and Black Bean Chili

Nutritional Information:

> ➢ Calories: 350 kcal
> ➢ Carbohydrates: 58g
> ➢ Protein: 14g
> ➢ Fat: 7g

Ingredients:

> ➢ 2 sweet potatoes, diced

- ➢ 1 can black beans, drained
- ➢ 1 can diced tomatoes
- ➢ 1 tbsp chili powder
- ➢ 2 cups vegetable broth

Preparation:

- ➢ In a pot, combine sweet potatoes, black beans, tomatoes, chili powder, and vegetable broth. Simmer until sweet potatoes are cooked through.

6. Spinach and Feta Omelette

Nutritional Information:

- ➢ Calories: 280 kcal
- ➢ Carbohydrates: 6g
- ➢ Protein: 20g
- ➢ Fat: 18g

Ingredients:

- ➢ 3 eggs
- ➢ 1 cup fresh spinach
- ➢ 2 tbsp crumbled feta cheese
- ➢ Salt and pepper to taste

Preparation:

- ➢ Beat eggs and pour into a heated skillet.
- ➢ Add spinach and feta. Cook until eggs are set. Fold the omelette and serve.

7. Lentil and Vegetable Soup

Nutritional Information:

- ➢ Calories: 260 kcal
- ➢ Carbohydrates: 45g
- ➢ Protein: 15g
- ➢ Fat: 3g

Ingredients:

- ➢ 1 cup lentils
- ➢ 2 carrots, chopped
- ➢ 1 onion, diced
- ➢ 4 cups vegetable broth

Preparation:

- ➢ In a pot, combine lentils, carrots, onion, and vegetable broth. Simmer until the lentils are tender.

8. Greek Yogurt Parfait with Berries and Nuts

Nutritional Information:

- ➢ Calories: 280 kcal
- ➢ Carbohydrates: 35g
- ➢ Protein: 15g
- ➢ Fat: 10g

Ingredients:

- ➢ 1 cup Greek yogurt
- ➢ ½ cup mixed berries
- ➢ 2 tbsp mixed nuts
- ➢ 1 tsp honey (optional)

Preparation:

> ➢ Arrange nuts, berries, and Greek yogurt in a glass.
> Drizzle with honey if desired.

9. Tofu and Broccoli Stir-Fry

Nutritional Information:

> ➢ Calories: 290 kcal
> ➢ Carbohydrates: 20g
> ➢ Protein: 22g
> ➢ Fat: 14g

Ingredients:

> ➢ 1 block tofu, cubed
> ➢ 2 cups broccoli florets
> ➢ 3 tbsp soy sauce
> ➢ 2 tbsp sesame oil

Preparation:

> ➢ Sauté tofu and broccoli in sesame oil.
> ➢ Add soy sauce and stir until evenly coated.

10. Cauliflower Rice Bowl with Grilled Chicken

Nutritional Information:

> ➢ Calories: 330 kcal
> ➢ Carbohydrates: 20g
> ➢ Protein: 30g
> ➢ Fat: 15g

Ingredients:

- ➢ 1 cup cauliflower rice
- ➢ 1 grilled chicken breast
- ➢ 1 cup mixed vegetables
- ➢ 2 tbsp teriyaki sauce

Preparation:

- ➢ Sauté cauliflower rice and mixed vegetables.
- ➢ Serve with sliced grilled chicken breast, drizzled with teriyaki sauce.

11. Baked Stuffed Bell Peppers

Nutritional Information:

- ➢ Calories: 310 kcal
- ➢ Carbohydrates: 42g
- ➢ Protein: 18g
- ➢ Fat: 8g

Ingredients:

- ➢ 4 bell peppers, halved
- ➢ 1 cup quinoa
- ➢ 1 can black beans, drained
- ➢ 1 cup salsa

Preparation:

- ➢ As directed on the package, prepare the quinoa.
- ➢ Mix quinoa with black beans and salsa. Stuff the bell peppers.
- ➢ Bake until peppers are tender and filling is heated through.

12. Tuna and Avocado Salad

Nutritional Information:

- ➢ Calories: 290 kcal
- ➢ Carbohydrates: 12g
- ➢ Protein: 26g
- ➢ Fat: 16g

Ingredients:

- ➢ 1 can tuna, drained
- ➢ 1 avocado, cubed
- ➢ Mixed greens
- ➢ Balsamic vinaigrette

Preparation:

- ➢ Add a balsamic vinaigrette to mixed greens.
- ➢ Top with tuna and avocado.

13. Mushroom and Spinach Frittata

Nutritional Information:

- ➢ Calories: 260 kcal
- ➢ Carbohydrates: 8g
- ➢ Protein: 18g
- ➢ Fat: 16g

Ingredients:

- ➢ 6 eggs
- ➢ 1 cup sliced mushrooms
- ➢ 2 cups fresh spinach
- ➢ 1/2 cup shredded cheese

Preparation:

> Sauté mushrooms and spinach in an ovenproof skillet.
> Beat eggs and pour over the vegetables. Sprinkle with cheese.
> In order for the eggs to set, bake.

14. Broccoli and Edamame Salad

Nutritional Information:

> Calories: 230 kcal
> Carbohydrates: 18g
> Protein: 14g
> Fat: 12g

Ingredients:

> 2 cups broccoli florets
> 1 cup shelled edamame
> 2 tbsp olive oil
> 1 tbsp lemon juice

Preparation:

> Steam broccoli and edamame until tender-crisp.
> Toss with olive oil and lemon juice.

15. Chia Seed Pudding with Berries

Nutritional Information:

> Calories: 280 kcal
> Carbohydrates: 30g
> Protein: 10g

➢ Fat: 15g

Ingredients:

➢ 1/4 cup chia seeds
➢ 1 cup almond milk
➢ 1 tsp honey
➢ Mixed berries

Preparation:

➢ Mix chia seeds and almond milk. Sweeten with honey if desired.
➢ Refrigerate until the mixture sets. Serve with mixed berries.

16. Grilled Shrimp and Zucchini Skewers

Nutritional Information:

➢ Calories: 250 kcal
➢ Carbohydrates: 12g
➢ Protein: 30g
➢ Fat: 10g

Ingredients:

➢ 12 big shrimp with deveined shells
➢ 2 zucchinis, sliced
➢ 2 tbsp olive oil
➢ 2 tsp Italian seasoning

Preparation:

➢ Toss shrimp and zucchini with olive oil and Italian seasoning.

> ➢ Thread onto skewers and grill until shrimp is pink and zucchini is tender.

17. Stuffed Portobello Mushrooms

Nutritional Information:

> ➢ Calories: 320 kcal
> ➢ Carbohydrates: 18g
> ➢ Protein: 15g
> ➢ Fat: 20g

Ingredients:

> ➢ 4 large portobello mushrooms
> ➢ 1 cup cooked quinoa
> ➢ 1 cup baby spinach
> ➢ 1/2 cup shredded mozzarella cheese

Preparation:

> ➢ Preheat oven to 375°F (190°C).
> ➢ Place mushrooms on a baking sheet. Divide quinoa, spinach, and cheese among the mushrooms.
> ➢ Bake until mushrooms are tender and filling is heated through.

18. Stir-Fried Tofu with Cashews and Broccoli

Nutritional Information:

> ➢ Calories: 290 kcal
> ➢ Carbohydrates: 22g
> ➢ Protein: 16g
> ➢ Fat: 18g

Ingredients:

- ➤ 1 block firm tofu, cubed
- ➤ 2 cups broccoli florets
- ➤ 1/2 cup roasted cashews
- ➤ 3 tbsp soy sauce

Preparation:

- ➤ In a pan, sauté the broccoli and tofu.
- ➤ Add soy sauce and cashews. Stir until the coating on the tofu is uniform.

Berry and Almond Smoothie Bowl

Nutritional Information:

- ➤ Calories: 320 kcal
- ➤ Carbohydrates: 40g
- ➤ Protein: 15g
- ➤ Fat: 12g

Ingredients:

- ➤ 1 cup mixed berries
- ➤ 1 ripe banana
- ➤ 1/4 cup almond butter
- ➤ 1/2 cup almond milk

Preparation:

- ➤ Blend berries, banana, almond butter, and almond milk until smooth. Pour into a bowl and top with sliced almonds and extra berries.

20. Mediterranean Tuna Salad Wrap

Nutritional Information:

- ➢ Calories: 340 kcal
- ➢ Carbohydrates: 22g
- ➢ Protein: 25g
- ➢ Fat: 18g

Ingredients:

- ➢ 1 can tuna, drained
- ➢ 1/4 cup diced cucumber
- ➢ 2 tbsp plain Greek yogurt
- ➢ 1 whole-grain wrap

Preparation:

- ➢ Mix tuna, cucumber, and Greek yogurt.
- ➢ Spoon the mixture onto the wrap, roll it up, and enjoy.

The recipes provided here are tailored to support hormonal health for women over 50. Each dish is carefully crafted to provide the essential nutrients required for hormonal balance while offering a variety of flavors, textures, and nutritional benefits. By incorporating these recipes into your diet, you can take proactive steps toward harmonizing your hormones and supporting overall well-being.

Chapter 8: Lifestyle Tips for Hormonal Wellness

This chapter is a crucial part of the book **Intermittent Fasting for Hormonal Balance in Women Over 50**, focusing on science-backed strategies for PMS relief, perimenopause harmony, and weight management. In this chapter, we will explore comprehensive, narrative-based, educative, descriptive, informative, engaging, actionable, supportive, and scientifically backed content tailored to women over 50 to promote hormonal wellness and overall well-being.

Lifestyle plays a significant role in hormonal balance, especially for women experiencing the natural hormonal shifts associated with aging. As we explore this chapter, we will discuss key lifestyle factors such as stress management, exercise, sleep, and mindfulness techniques to support hormonal wellness. Additionally, we will delve into actionable lifestyle changes and habits that can provide essential support for hormonal balance.

Stress Management for Hormonal Wellness

Women over 50 often face high levels of stress due to various personal, professional, and family responsibilities. Chronic stress can significantly impact hormonal balance, leading to symptoms such as fatigue, mood swings, and disrupted sleep patterns. Therefore, incorporating stress management techniques into daily life is vital for hormonal wellness.

Actionable Tips for Stress Management

- Practice mindfulness and meditation: Engaging in regular mindfulness practices, such as meditation and deep breathing exercises, can help reduce stress levels and promote hormonal balance.

- Time management and prioritization: Organizing daily tasks and scheduling time for relaxation and self-care can reduce stress and support overall well-being.

- Connecting with nature: Spending time in nature, whether through walks in the park or gardening, can have a calming effect on the mind and body, promoting hormonal balance.

Exercise for Hormonal Balance

Regular physical activity is essential for overall health and plays a crucial role in supporting hormonal balance. As women age, maintaining an active lifestyle becomes increasingly important for managing hormonal changes and promoting overall well-being.

Effective Exercise Strategies

- Strength training: Incorporating strength training exercises into your routine can help maintain muscle mass, support bone health, and contribute to hormonal balance.

- Aerobic exercise: Engaging in aerobic activities like walking, swimming, or dancing can enhance cardiovascular health and improve hormonal regulation.

- Flexibility exercises: Practicing yoga or stretching exercises can help maintain flexibility, reduce muscle tension, and support overall well-being.

Quality Sleep for Hormonal Wellness

Sleep is fundamental for hormonal balance and overall health, yet many women over 50 struggles with insomnia, disrupted sleep patterns, and other sleep-related issues. Prioritizing quality sleep is essential to support hormonal wellness and overall vitality.

Guidelines for Improving Sleep Quality

- Establishing a consistent sleep schedule: Going to bed and waking up at the same time each day can regulate the body's internal clock, promoting better sleep quality.
- Creating a restful sleep environment: Ensure your bedroom is conducive to quality sleep by minimizing noise, light, and electronic distractions.
- Practicing relaxation techniques: Engaging in relaxation practices such as gentle stretching, reading, or listening to soothing music before bedtime can promote better sleep.

Mindfulness and Hormonal Balance

Incorporating mindfulness practices into daily life can have significant benefits for hormonal wellness. Mindfulness techniques can help manage stress, promote emotional health, and support overall hormonal balance.

Practical Mindfulness Tips

- Mindful eating: Paying attention to the sensory experience of eating, such as taste, texture, and aroma, can enhance the enjoyment of meals and support healthy eating habits.

- Gratitude journaling: Taking time to acknowledge and appreciate positive aspects of daily life through gratitude journaling can cultivate a positive mindset and reduce stress.

Incorporating these lifestyle tips into daily routines can provide essential support for hormonal wellness among women over 50. By implementing stress management strategies, engaging in regular exercise, prioritizing quality sleep, and cultivating mindfulness, women can empower themselves to navigate the natural effects of hormonal changes with resilience and vitality.

Importance of Exercise in Hormonal Balance

The presence of hormonal imbalance is a common concern for many women over 50. These imbalances can lead to a variety of symptoms, including weight gain, mood swings, hot flashes, and more. Integrating a balanced diet, exercise, and lifestyle adjustments can significantly help in managing hormonal balance. In this chapter, we will explore the crucial role of exercise in achieving hormonal balance. We will discuss how different forms of exercise impact hormones and delve into specific types of exercises that can be particularly beneficial for women over 50.

The Impact of Exercise on Hormonal Balance

Regular physical activity has a profound impact on hormonal balance, especially in women over 50. Exercise helps to regulate the production and functioning of hormones, which in turn can alleviate symptoms associated with menopause, PMS, and other hormonal imbalances.

1. Regulation of Insulin

As individuals age, insulin sensitivity tends to decrease, making it harder for the body to regulate blood sugar levels. This can lead to weight gain and an increased risk of developing conditions like type 2 diabetes. Engaging in regular physical activity, particularly resistance training and endurance exercises, can enhance insulin sensitivity, effectively managing blood sugar levels and reducing the risk of insulin-related imbalances.

2. Influence on Estrogen Levels

Estrogen plays a pivotal role in various bodily functions, and its decline during menopause can lead to several symptoms. Engaging in weight-bearing exercises such as strength training and weightlifting can help maintain bone density, minimizing the risk of osteoporosis, which is especially important for women over 50. Moreover, some research suggests that regular physical activity may help moderate estrogen levels, which could alleviate symptoms associated with menopause.

3. Regulation of Cortisol

Chronic stress can result in elevated cortisol levels, which, when sustained, can contribute to hormonal imbalances. Regular exercise both reduces overall stress levels and helps manage cortisol productin. Engaging in activities like yoga, Pilates, or moderate aerobic exercise can be particularly effective in lowering stress and soothing the nervous system.

4. Impact on Thyroid Function

Regular physical activity can help optimize thyroid function, potentially benefitting women dealing with thyroid imbalances. It is important to note that excessive or intense exercise may negatively impact thyroid health, particularly in individuals with existing thyroid conditions. Therefore, moderation is key when it comes to managing thyroid health through exercise.

Types of Exercises for Hormonal Balance

When it comes to exercise specifically catered to hormonal balance in women over 50, it's important to consider a holistic approach that incorporates elements of cardio, strength training, flexibility, and stress-reducing activities.

1. Cardiovascular Exercise

Engaging in cardiovascular activities such as brisk walking, cycling, swimming, or dancing not only promotes heart health but also supports weight management and improves overall mood. Regular cardiovascular exercise has been linked to improved circulation, reduced stress, and enhanced endurance, making it a vital component of hormonal balance for women over 50.

2. Strength Training

Incorporating strength training exercises into your routine is essential for maintaining muscle mass and bone density. As women age, there is a natural decline in muscle mass, which can contribute to a slower metabolism and reduced strength. Resistance training using weights, resistance bands, or bodyweight exercises can help counteract these effects and promote hormonal balance.

3. Yoga and Pilates

Activities like yoga and Pilates not only contribute to flexibility and core strength but also have a profound impact on stress reduction. These mind-body practices can help regulate cortisol levels and bring a sense of calm and balance, making them particularly beneficial for women dealing with hormonal fluctuations.

4. Flexibility Training

Maintaining flexibility becomes increasingly important with age. Incorporating activities that focus on flexibility, such as stretching, tai chi, or gentle movement exercises, can help improve joint health, posture, and overall mobility, contributing to a well-rounded exercise routine for women over 50.

Customizing an Exercise Routine for Hormonal Balance

When designing an exercise routine tailored to hormonal balance, it's crucial to consider individual preferences, fitness levels, and any underlying health conditions. Starting slowly and gradually increasing the intensity and duration of exercise can help prevent injury and support long-term adherence to a workout regimen.

Engaging in activities that are enjoyable and fulfilling is key to maintaining consistency. Understanding the need for variety in a workout routine can help keep things interesting and prevent boredom or plateauing. Additionally, focusing on holistic wellness, including adequate rest and recovery, is essential in achieving hormonal balance through exercise.

In conclusion, exercise plays a pivotal role in managing hormonal balance for women over 50. By incorporating a diverse range of physical activities and exercising in moderation, women can alleviate symptoms associated with hormonal imbalances and support overall health and well-being. Customizing an exercise routine to individual needs while emphasizing a balanced approach to various forms of exercise can greatly contribute to hormonal wellness.

Stress Management Techniques

As women navigate the transformative years beyond 50, hormonal fluctuations coupled with the challenges of everyday life can often lead to increased stress levels. This, in turn, can impact overall well-being, including hormonal balance. In the pursuit of a harmonious and healthy life, it is crucial to embrace effective stress management techniques. In this chapter, we will delve into scientifically-backed strategies to manage stress, nurture hormonal equilibrium, and promote overall well-being for women over 50.

The Impact of Stress on Hormonal Balance

Before delving into stress management techniques, it is vital to understand the intricate relationship between stress and hormonal balance in the female body. As individuals experience stress, the body's natural response triggers the release of cortisol, often referred to as the "stress hormone." While cortisol plays a crucial role in the body's fight-or-flight response, sustained high levels of cortisol due to chronic stress can disrupt the delicate balance of other hormones such as estrogen and progesterone, leading to a range of adverse effects, including irregular menstrual cycles, exacerbation of menopausal symptoms, and increased susceptibility to conditions like osteoporosis and heart disease.

In the context of intermittent fasting for hormonal balance, addressing stress becomes paramount, as the overall goal is to create an environment conducive to hormonal harmony and overall well-being. By incorporating stress management techniques into one's routine, women over 50 can support their endocrine system, alleviate menopausal symptoms, and foster a sense of balance in their daily lives.

Empowering Stress Management Techniques

1. Mindfulness Meditation: Cultivating a regular mindfulness meditation practice can be immensely beneficial in managing stress. For women over 50, mindfulness meditation offers a powerful tool to quiet the mind, reduce anxiety, and enhance emotional resilience. Scientific studies have shown that mindfulness practices can lower cortisol levels, improve sleep patterns, and foster a greater sense of well-being. Encouraging women to integrate mindfulness into their daily routine can lead to profound reductions in stress and contribute to hormonal equilibrium.

2. Physical Activity and Exercise: Engaging in regular physical activity and exercise is a cornerstone of stress management for women over 50. Exercise acts as a potent stress-reducer, promoting the release of endorphins, which are natural mood lifters. From brisk walking and yoga to strength training, women can explore a diverse range of physical activities that resonate with their preferences and lifestyle. By doing so, they not only manage stress but also support hormonal balance, bone health, and overall vitality.

3. Nutrition and Meal Planning: Proper nutrition is a fundamental component of stress management. Encouraging women to adopt a balanced, whole-food diet that supports hormonal balance and includes adequate sources of nutrients like omega-3 fatty acids, magnesium, and vitamin C can significantly impact stress

levels. Meal planning can introduce a sense of structure and empowerment, fostering a positive relationship with food and promoting overall well-being.

4. Quality Sleep: Adequate and restorative sleep is essential for managing stress and nurturing hormonal balance. Encouraging women to prioritize sleep hygiene, establish calming bedtime rituals, and create a tranquil sleep environment can enhance the quality of their rest. Scientific evidence indicates that sufficient sleep contributes to reduced stress levels, improved cognitive function, and overall well-being.

5. Social Support and Connection: Cultivating and nurturing genuine social connections can provide vital emotional support for women over 50. Building a network of friends, engaging in shared activities, and seeking support from like-minded individuals can mitigate the impact of stress on hormonal balance. Research illustrates that social interactions and support systems play a pivotal role in buffering the effects of stress and promoting emotional resilience.

Integrating Stress Management with Intermittent Fasting

In the context of "Intermittent Fasting for Hormonal Balance in Women Over 50," the integration of stress management techniques is instrumental. By embracing these strategies, women can empower themselves to navigate the transformative years with resilience, grace, and a profound sense of well-being. As women cultivate mindfulness, engage in physical activity, embrace nourishing nutrition, prioritize quality sleep, and foster meaningful connections, they embark on a transformative journey that not only supports hormonal balance but also nurtures the essence of holistic health.

In conclusion, the adoption of stress management techniques is indispensable in nurturing hormonal balance for women over 50. By grounding these strategies in scientific insight and practical application, women can embark on a journey of empowerment, resilience, and vitality. As they navigate the transformative landscape of perimenopause and beyond, the fusion of stress management and intermittent fasting sets the stage for profound well-being, hormonal harmony, and a life enriched by balance and grace.

Quality Sleep and Its Impact on Hormones

For women over 50, the interplay between hormones and overall health becomes increasingly critical. During this phase of life, hormonal shifts can lead to various challenges such as PMS symptoms, perimenopause, and weight management issues. In the pursuit of holistic wellness, one often overlooked yet profoundly impactful aspect is the quality of sleep and its influence on hormonal balance. In this chapter, we'll delve into the significance of quality sleep and its direct impact on hormonal equilibrium in women over 50. By understanding this vital relationship, we can unlock strategies for enhancing sleep quality and, in turn, support optimal hormonal health.

The Importance of Quality Sleep for Women Over 50

As women navigate through their 50s and beyond, the significance of quality sleep should not be underestimated. Sleep is the cornerstone of well-being, with its restorative effects impacting not only energy levels and cognitive function but also the delicate balance of hormones within the body. Adequate, restful sleep is inherently linked to the regulation of key hormones that play a central role in women's health, including estrogen, progesterone, cortisol, and growth hormone.

Hormonal Balance and Sleep Patterns

The relationship between sleep and hormonal balance is intricate and multifaceted. One of the primary hormones affected by sleep is cortisol, often referred to as the body's stress hormone. Inadequate or poor-quality sleep can lead to dysregulated cortisol levels, resulting in heightened stress responses and potential disruptions to other hormones, ultimately impacting overall well-being. Furthermore, irregular sleep patterns can influence the production of growth hormone, a key player in tissue repair, muscle growth, and the maintenance of healthy body composition. Sleep disturbances can hinder the release of growth hormone, potentially affecting metabolic processes.

Estrogen and Progesterone Regulation

In the context of women's health, the impact of sleep on estrogen and progesterone levels is noteworthy. Quality sleep contributes to the balanced regulation of these hormones, supporting menstrual regularity and overall hormonal equilibrium. Sleep disturbances can disrupt the delicate interplay between estrogen and progesterone, potentially leading to irregular menstrual cycles and exacerbating perimenopausal symptoms. Understanding the pivotal role of sleep in estrogen and progesterone modulation fosters an appreciation for the profound influence of quality sleep on women's hormonal well-being.

Strategies for Enhancing Sleep Quality

Recognizing the pivotal role of quality sleep in hormonal balance underscores the importance of implementing effective strategies to enhance sleep quality for women over 50. Here, we explore actionable techniques aimed at improving sleep patterns and overall well-being:

1. Establishing a Consistent Sleep Schedule: Encouraging a regular sleep schedule reinforces the body's internal clock, promoting a sense of balance within the hormonal system.

2. Creating a Restful Sleep Environment: Optimizing the sleep environment by minimizing light exposure, reducing noise, and ensuring comfortable bedding can facilitate deeper, more restorative sleep.

3. Prioritizing Relaxation Techniques: Engaging in relaxation practices such as meditation, deep breathing exercises, or gentle yoga before bedtime can calm the mind and prepare the body for restful sleep.

4. Nurturing Daily Physical Activity: Regular physical activity plays a significant role in promoting healthy sleep patterns, enhancing overall well-being, and contributing to hormonal balance.

5. Embracing Mindfulness Practices: Cultivating mindfulness through activities like journaling, gratitude exercises, and mindfulness meditation can alleviate stress, fostering an environment that is conducive to better sleep.

6. Evaluating Dietary Choices: Mindful consumption of sleep-promoting foods and the avoidance of stimulating substances like caffeine and alcohol close to bedtime can positively impact sleep quality.

7. Seeking Professional Guidance: In cases where sleep disturbances persist, consulting healthcare professionals,

such as sleep specialists or healthcare providers, can provide valuable insights and personalized strategies for addressing specific sleep challenges.

Furthermore, the implementation of intermittent fasting, as discussed in this book, has been shown to have positive effects on sleep patterns and hormonal balance. By incorporating intermittent fasting strategies in alignment with individual needs and preferences, women over 50 can further support their quest for quality sleep and harmonious hormonal health.

In the pursuit of hormonal balance and overall well-being, women over 50 must recognize the profound impact of quality sleep on their health. Understanding the intricate relationship between sleep and hormonal regulation equips women with the knowledge and strategies necessary to support optimal sleep patterns and hormonal equilibrium. By prioritizing restful sleep and implementing actionable techniques to enhance sleep quality, women can embark on a journey towards holistic well-being, empowered by the transformative influence of quality sleep on hormonal balance.

Conclusion

After an extensive journey exploring the ins and outs of hormonal balance through intermittent fasting, it's time to reflect on the invaluable insights we've garnered along the way. The **Intermittent Fasting for Hormonal Balance in Women Over 50** has empowered us to delve deeper into the realm of PMS relief, perimenopause harmony, weight management, and hormone-balancing success. As we conclude this chapter, let's embrace the key takeaways and revelations that have the potential to revolutionize our well-being.

Throughout this comprehensive guide, we've unfolded the science-backed strategies that resonate with the specific needs of women over 50. It's been a narratively captivating journey into exploring the impact of intermittent fasting on hormonal balance and how it can manifest in PMS relief, perimenopause harmony, and effective weight management. The delightful meal plans and easy recipes have not only tantalized our taste buds but also provided a crucial foundation for sustaining these scientifically supported strategies.

At the heart of this conclusion lies the understanding that managing hormonal balance isn't a one-size-fits-all solution. As women over 50, we navigate a unique and dynamic landscape of hormonal changes. What is effective for one person might not have the same effect on another. Therefore, our collective pursuit of hormone balance must be rooted in personalized experimentation and an unwavering commitment to discovering what truly works for our bodies.

The book has shed light on the significance of incorporating intermittent fasting into our lifestyles. This approach, when tailored to our individual needs, stands as a powerful tool to regulate and optimize hormonal fluctuations. As women in this pivotal phase of life, the impact of hormone balance transcends beyond the physical realm. It influences our emotional well-being, our vitality, and our overall quality of life.

Furthermore, the educational aspect of this journey has been enlightening—empowering us with a deep understanding of the intricate interplay between intermittent fasting, hormonal dynamics, and the profound implications it holds for our bodies. Embracing the science-backed strategies and integrating them into our daily routines has the potential to bring about transformative change, allowing us to reclaim agency over our health and well-being.

As we draw the curtains on this book, let's not forget the actionable insights we've unearthed. Implementing intermittent fasting with a focus on hormonal balance demands dedication, patience, and an open mindset toward adapting to the unique signals our bodies convey. Through the consistent application of these strategies, we're not only fostering a harmonious relationship with our hormones but also nurturing a newfound sense of empowerment.

In closing, the culmination of our journey through "Intermittent Fasting for Hormonal Balance in Women Over 50" fosters a deep sense of optimism and potential. The takeaway isn't merely a collection of scientific insights and meal plans; it's the affirmation of our ability to take charge of our well-being. The conclusion encapsulates the beginning of a transformative path—one that promises PMS relief, perimenopause harmony, weight management, and the overarching success of balancing our hormones.

In this conclusion, we recognize that our individual explorations will continue—imbued with the knowledge gained and the momentum to move forward with confidence. Let this be the launching pad for a future marked by vitality, resilience, and the unwavering commitment to nurturing the hormone balance that supports our holistic well-being.